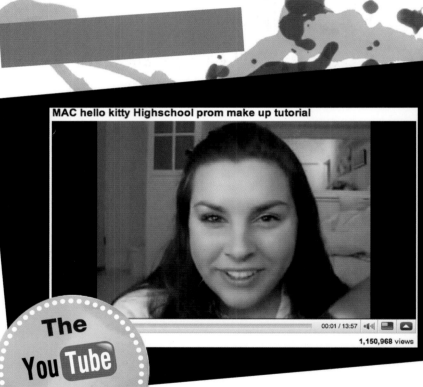

MAC hello kitty Highschool prom make up tutorial

00:01 / 13:57

1,150,968 views

The You Tube Sensation

Lauren ☺

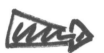

LAUREN LUKE LOOKS

25 CELEBRITY AND EVERYDAY MAKEUP TUTORIALS

LAUREN LUKE

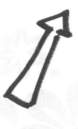

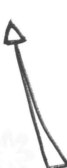

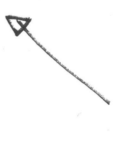

A FIRESIDE BOOK
Published by Simon & Schuster
New York London Toronto Sydney

Fireside
A Division of Simon & Schuster, Inc.
1230 Avenue of the Americas
New York, NY 10020

First Fireside trade paperback edition March 2010

FIRESIDE and colophon are registered trademarks
of Simon & Schuster, Inc.

For information about special discounts for bulk purchases,
please contact Simon & Schuster Special Sales at 1-866-506-1949
or business@simonandschuster.com.

The Simon & Schuster Speakers Bureau can bring authors to your
live event. For more information or to book an event contact the
Simon & Schuster Speakers Bureau at 1-866-248-3049 or visit our
website at www.simonspeakers.com.

Manufactured in the United States of America

10 9 8 7 6 5 4 3 2 1

Library of Congress Cataloging-in-Publication data is available.

ISBN 978-1-4391-8730-2

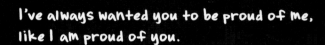

I've always wanted you to be proud of me, like I am proud of you.

Times haven't always been easy for either of us, but you have always been understanding, despite your young age, of all the times I have had to spend away from you working to secure our futures. Considering the circumstances of raising you alone at such a young age, I feel very lucky to have such a good boy. You are a gem!

It's nice seeing you grow and stand on your own two feet and become a best friend to me. You are my little man, but you're not too big to hold my hand in public even though you might think otherwise!

CONTENTS

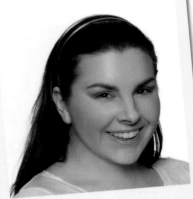

Sweet & innocent

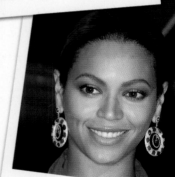

Vintage gold

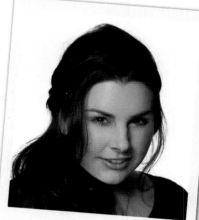

Rosebud beauty

How to choose the right colors for you
Paint box

page 36

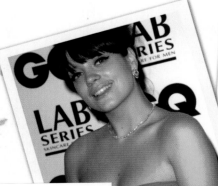

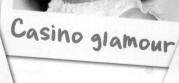

Casino glamour

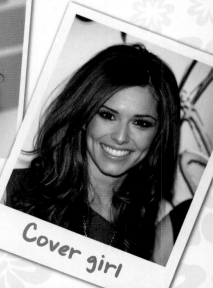

Cover girl

THIS IS WHO I AM
MY STORY

My story really should start "Once upon a time"...I honestly do feel like I am living a fairy tale. The beginning of the story would describe the hard knock events of childhood. The wicked witch would probably take many forms, most of them characters from my school days. I would play the unfortunate princess and call myself Princess LaLa (a name given to me by my mam). Princess LaLa would strive and struggle and one day be rewarded when she met her handsome prince who would take her away and she would live happily ever after...

Most of this is true, except the handsome prince left on some quest of a single life once he became a father and the real savior of this story were the millions of little princes and princesses who watched me on their computer screens from bedrooms across the world.

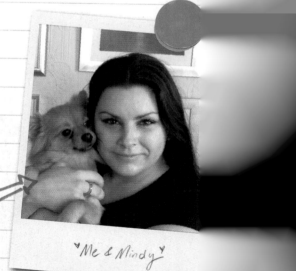

"Me & Mindy"

ISN'T SHE SO CUTE!!

THIS IS HOW IT ALL HAPPENED.

I was born in South Shields and have lived there in the same house with my family all my life. Living in the northeast of England is pretty tough for many, but I think it's fair to say our family had less money to go around than most. In hindsight, this isn't a bad thing. I certainly struggled with poverty while growing up (girls have an image to keep up, especially princesses), but I do feel that I can fully appreciate the finer things that have come my way in recent times. My past helps me to stay real and keep my feet on the ground.

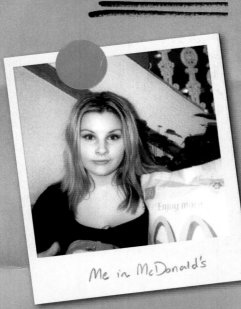

Me in McDonald's

My school years were a nightmare. I never seemed to fit in. I was far too distracted trying to avoid the school bullies to actually spend time learning anything from the teachers who seemed to ignore my plight. I have been told more than once that I wouldn't amount to anything. I had no friends to speak of at school, so for the most part it was a lonely and frightening experience.

When my sister Helen came along I had a friend to play with at last. We used to get up to so much mischief around our house, it's a wonder we didn't drive our parents crazy! I have always been creative, and from a very young age I would think nothing of experimenting with crayons, melting them onto the radiators because I liked the colors and the effect it created.

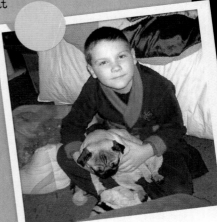

♥ Jordan & Phoebe

I would create concoctions from all manner of tubes, pots, and jars and could regularly be found mixing toothpaste and jam with anything I could get my hands on. I liked the colors, but I don't think my parents shared my viewpoint.

Helen and I created our own nonsense language, which was made up of funny accents and snippets of things we would hear on TV or playing computer games. This is actually where "zoom, zoom" came from. The characters of the computer game The Sims would say good-bye with something that sounded like "soom, soom" and Helen and I changed it and made it our own. It seems to have stuck with me because I regularly sign off my videos with "Zoom, zoom!"

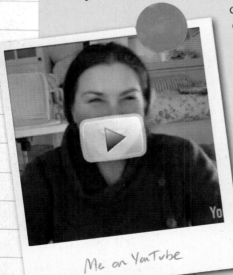

Little Me at my desk

Two more sisters arrived when I was thirteen. Twins Rachel and Mikayla were born premature, weighing just 1 lb. 6 oz. and 1 lb. 12 oz., and we were told neither was likely to survive. They really were miracle babies because they defied the doctors and chose to live. Despite a few learning difficulties which they handle brilliantly, they are now both enjoying teenage life and all the thrills that come with it.

Not long after their birth I was enjoying my own teenage thrills, and despite my lack of popularity at school, I managed to start dating. About six months into our relationship when I was fifteen years old I lost my virginity to Jordan's father. I was lying there watching Felix the Cat on TV, thinking to myself that I was having

Me on YouTube

sex and feeling that all the curiosity preceding sex didn't match the feelings discovered during the actual event. So much of my innocence was lost that day, soon to be replaced with the hard realities that accompany being pregnant at fifteen.

I dropped out of school early because of the pregnancy and gave birth to Jordan when I was sixteen. Jordan's father decided he wasn't willing to play mammies and daddies and left me a few days later. I was heartbroken. I wondered how I was going to manage to raise Jordan on my pocket money. I really didn't have a clue.

Soon afterwards, my dad left to go his own way, too, and my parents got divorced.

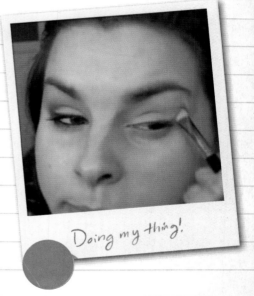

Doing my thing!

There I was with a baby on my knee, my mam with her own troubles trying to cope on her own with the young twins. We sat together on the settee laughing and crying at the madness of it all. My fate could have easily been sealed there and then, but I still had the feeling in the back of my mind that it could be different.

I decided I needed a job. I took volunteer work at a local charity shop to get some retail experience and worked there for around six months before I quit to work in a newsagent's shop. I stayed there for about eighteen months before taking another job as a barmaid in a local pub. I hated it, but I needed the money. After working in the bar for a couple of years I then took work as a taxi dispatcher. The pay was slightly better and the hours were more suited to raising my son.

About four years into my taxi job I decided I needed something with better prospects for Jordan and me. We were barely getting by, and I wanted a more secure future for the both of us.

I've always enjoyed using and experimenting with makeup and looked into setting up my own business on eBay selling cosmetics.

I didn't really have much spare cash to start a business, but I managed to put a small amount aside to buy my first batch of stock. Orders were slow at first, but I gradually built it up enough so that I could leave my job in the taxi office and devote more time to Jordan and my little business—which I ran from my bedroom.

Things eventually started to take off, and I had—for the first time in my life—a regular income from a job that I enjoyed doing.

As the orders came in, I used to get quite a few requests asking how some of the products should best be applied and which colors would suit certain eye or hair colors. I used to reply to all of these questions by e-mail, but eventually there were so many requests that I couldn't keep up with them and run my business properly.

I then discovered an Internet site called YouTube where you could upload short videos and everyone could watch them. I thought this was great and decided to start making short tutorials about the products I was using and then sending people the link so they could watch. I was a little bit nervous at first and only expected a handful of people to watch them—I mean I wasn't even a qualified makeup artist and was completely self-taught.

It didn't take long before people started to watch and then watch in the hundreds and then thousands. I was blown away and couldn't believe so many people wanted to watch me in my bedroom showing people how to put on makeup.

Requests for certain looks started flooding in and, when I made a video where I showed people how to re-create the Leona Lewis look that she wore in her "Bleeding Love" video, things just went berserk, and all of a sudden I had millions of people watching my videos.

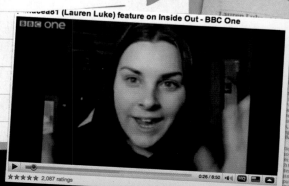

HOW si
her be

(Lauren Luke) feature on Inside Out - BBC One
BBC one

★★★★★ 2,087 ratings   0:26 / 8:50

The Look

LAUREN LUKE
FLAWLESS FOUNDATION

1 Start with a clean and moisturised face to create a soft, even base. Apply foundation to face and eyes. Mac's face and body foundation is great for hiding imperfections. Apply with a brush rather than fingers - it looks smoother and bonds to your moisturiser, so lasts longer.

2 On to your flawless canvas now build colour. I like Boots No7 skin highlights in peach, and it's ideal for glowing winter skin. Dab to the high of your cheek and up to your temple, then to the forehead and down your nose to achieve the effect of natural light catching your skin.

3 Now add a bronzer - great for contouring the side of your face if it looks a bit plump. Add to any part that you want to shadow out. For a more hollow-cheeked appearance, use a brush and stroke away from cheek up to hairline. Use under chin to make this area look slimmer, too.

4 Finish with light to medium pink cream blush. My favourite is by make-up artist Paula Dorf - her cheek colour creme in 'Playmate' is a fresh and perky shade. Apply with a brush for a long-lasting effect. Add clear lip gloss or good old Vaseline and you're ready for any weather.

Lauren Luke's make-up tutorials, filmed in her bedroom in South Shields, have attracted more than 26 million hits on YouTube. You can see a video of this look at guardian.co.uk/video

25 March 2009
Accessibility help
Text only

Homepage
Inside Out
England

Inside Out

Inside Out
North East

You are in: Inside Out > North East > Make-up guru

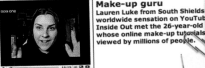
A video-star is born!

Make-up guru
Lauren Luke from South Shields worldwide sensation on YouTube Inside Out met the 26-year-old whose online make-up tutorials viewed by millions of people.

Lauren has developed her own type of celebrity influenced styles.

She's shown her viewers how their appearance of stars, from Miley Cy

See Lauren's Amy Winehouse tr
The BBC is not responsible for the content of

And all the tutorials are among m YouTube channel... The Leona Le more than 2 million times.

And there's even a fan page set

See the Lauren fan site >
The BBC is not responsible for the conte

How it began

Lauren started selling eye-ma taking photos of the products w how they were appli

WordPress.com

Blogs about:

Luke - internat

CBS NEWS
March 25, 200

The Self-Made Makeup Mave
27-Year-Old U.K. Single Mother's Instructional Videos Draw 41
Unexpectant Celebrity

LONDON, Feb. 28, 2009 | by Eleanor Tuohy

E-MAIL STORY | PRINT STORY | SPHERE

(CBS)
This story was writte

Lauren Luke is on a f She's charming, direc what has happened to

If the name Lauren Lu are obviously not a tee user.

A little over two years a working evenings as a t local cab company, hati 10-year-old son.

Now she's a YouTube se due in stores worldwide a a book being published in idea started in her bedroo

Luke, a single mother livin sister, decided the time ha that would allow her to wor hours. She began selling m the business picked up, she makeup application on You saved her from typing up e-r customer questions.

That was when Lauren's life people started watching her v million viewers and Luke mov According to Luke, her videos

Lauren Luke, 27, is a single mother from Tyneside, England, whose YouTube videos on makeup application have made her an Internet sensation. **(YouTube)**

RELATED

PHOTO ESSAY
Celebrity Circuit
Zac Efron at Paris premiere; plus, Cate Blanchett, Audrina Patridge, Tina Fey and Kevin James

STORIES
- YouTubers Caught in Warner Music Spat
- Pope Launches YouTube Channel

channel, pancea81, has drawn more than 4.5 second-most watched YouTube slots in Britain. hits worldwide.

The turning point, Luke says, was when she posted a tutorial on how to recre up from her *Bleeding Love* music video.

"That's when things really started to go berserk," as she applies the make up to herself looking stra became a template for dozens more videos, each the videos demonstrate how to create celebrity loo

VANITY

SUBSCRIBE | CULTURE

VANITY FAIR

VF Daily's
SOCIETY
& STYLE

Blog

Tips? vfdaily@vf.com

VF Daily
Culture & Celebrity
Politics & Power
Society & Style
James Wolcott's Blog
Little Gold Men (Movies)

FEATURED POSTS

VA
T
by

rtisingAge®

More from Ad Age: Creativity AdAgeChina Bookstore Jobs Sign up for E-mail

Get a FREE insider's look at the latest eMarketer analysis.
Two new articles each weekday.

E-mail | License Content | Print | Comment | RSS

Stay on top of the news and stay ahead of the game—sign up for e-mail newsletters now!

From YouTube Videos to Your Makeup Bag

Anomaly Shepherds Cosmetics Line by Self-Made Maven
Luke to Market

Series: The look: Lauren Luke's makeup tutorials

Lauren Luke: 'Just steady your little finger and practise'

The YouTube makeup guru marvels at the global popularity her amateur how-to videos

Esther Addley
guardian.co.uk, Friday 30 January 2009 13.19 GMT
Article history

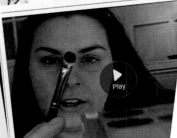
Play

mother giving make-up tips in
n became a global celebrity

lebrity. A 27-year-old single mother
lives with her 10-year-old son,
age nieces and five highly affectionate
ouse in an anonymous terraced street.

out of school early without

d, Charles is right...Lauren began selling makeup on eBay, and uploading
ompanying makeup tutorials to YouTube. It was these tutorials that caught the onlin
blics imagination. Lauren's YouTube channel, panacea81, has drawn more than 4.5
llion viewers and is one of the UK's most watched YouTube channels.

Web is driven by
age group

6 Oct 2008
The rise and rise of the
YouTube generation, and how adults can help

girl next chool -
at her local

amateur, who pursues activities to an increasingly important role in our society and

Vanaeas SUBSCRIBE

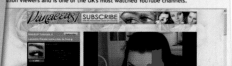

Newspapers and magazines started writing nice stories about me, and even TV stations were asking for an interview or wanting to make programs about me. It really is surreal. A lot of people ask what it's like to be a celebrity, but the truth is, I don't feel like one. I have had 50 million views on my YouTube channel so far, but I can't picture what 50 million people look like or ever hope to meet them all. I just turn on my camera and start recording myself putting makeup on, as I talk to my friends online. I have made quite a few good friends since this all started, and it's nice to finally feel like I am being spoken to without people looking down at me. This makes me feel happy, but I still don't feel like a celebrity.

I know what it's like to have no friends and no confidence, and I hope to make people feel better about themselves. Feeling OK in the head is more important than how much makeup we wear or how we wear it, but it can help us to feel a bit better about ourselves and boosts our confidence.

I do like trying out loud colors and wacky looks, but I also like to keep it real. I don't like the way traditional advertising for beauty and fashion uses only drop-dead gorgeous models or ultra-skinny girls. Most of us don't look like Kate Moss; I'm not even sure Kate Moss looks like Kate Moss without the clever photography and tinkering about with the lens and lighting. Don't get me wrong, I'm not mad at beautiful women or glamorous images, I just think there is a standard that is set by the industry that is unobtainable by the vast majority of us normal folk who pay for it. We are all entitled to have products that work and bring out the best in us and to create looks that we can actually wear.

So here I am with my own book of looks worn by little old me. Some looks are for fun or special occasions, and some of them for everyday use. I hope you like them, and I really hope you try some of them out. If you like them, then let me know. I'd love to hear from you. I hope you have as much fun trying them out as I did creating them for this book.

I have come to realize anything is possible if you try hard enough. When I was at school, I made the mistake of letting a few bullies in on my little secret desire to one day go to America and make something of myself. One day when coming out of school I noticed that they had painted a slogan on a wall I used to pass on my way home which read "Lauren's going to America, yeah right!"

On April 27, 2009, I launched my own makeup line in Times Square in New York City.

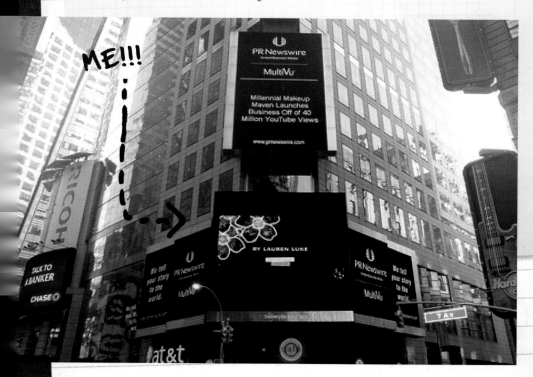

HAVE FAITH IN YOURSELF, AND IT WILL HAPPEN!

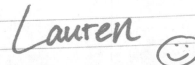

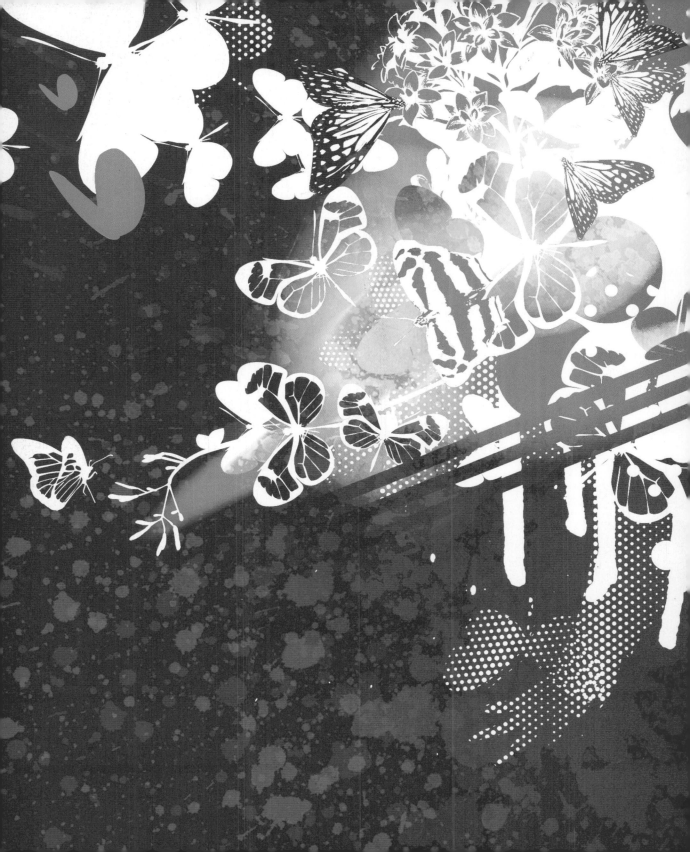

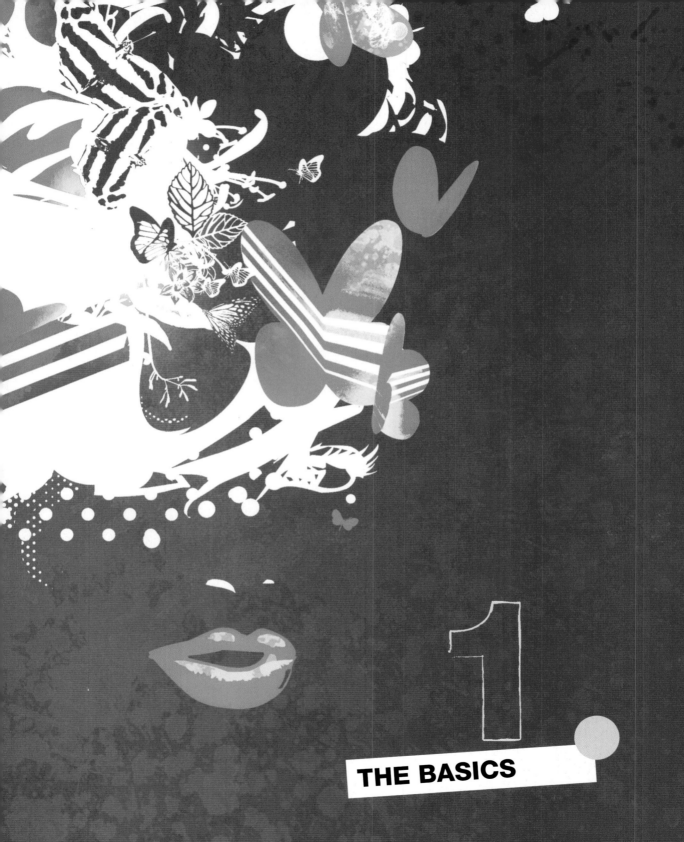

1.

THE BASICS

THIS IS ME

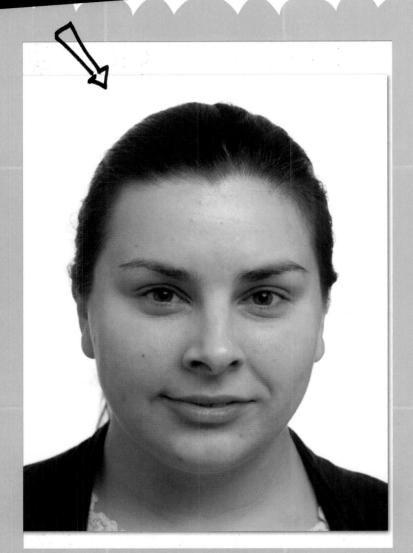

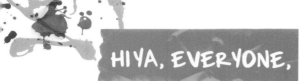

HIYA, EVERYONE,

Here's the real deal before any makeup—spots and imperfections, and all.

THE BLANK CANVAS.

In this section I am going to run through the basics which apply to all my looks such as primers, concealer, foundation, bronzer, blusher, highlighter, mascara, eyeliner, and the shape of your eyebrows, and I'm going to introduce you to what they do and how they can help you on your way to fabulous features.

I've learned lots of little tricks and techniques along the way, and I want to pass them on to you.

Lauren

SPEND TIME WITH YOURSELF

★ TAKE A BAG OF MAKEUP, SIT IN FRONT OF A MIRROR, AND JUST HAVE FUN

★ YOU'LL BE SURPRISED AT HOW HAPPY YOU FEEL GETTING TO KNOW YOUR OWN FACE

★ IT'S SO EASY TO GET INTO A RUT AND APPLY THE MAKEUP EVERYONE TELLS YOU TO

★ BY SITTING DOWN AND STARING AT YOURSELF IN THE MIRROR YOU CAN WORK OUT WHERE YOUR CHEEKBONES ARE AND WHERE TO SHADE AND HIGHLIGHT YOUR FACE— EVERYBODY IS DIFFERENT

★ WORK OUT HOW TO MAKE THE MOST OF YOUR BONE STRUCTURE BY VISUALIZING A 3-D GRAPH OVER YOUR FACE AND PLAYING AROUND WITH SHADING AND HIGHLIGHTING

★ MY EYES ARE MY BEST FEATURE. MY LIPS ARE NOT. SO I CONCENTRATE ON BRINGING OUT MY EYES AND USUALLY LEAVE MY LIPS NEUTRAL—AND THAT'S RIGHT FOR MY FACE

★ LEARN TO PLAY UP YOUR STRENGTHS AND DITCH THE REST. IT'S SILLY TO MAKE YOURSELF UNHAPPY FOR OTHERS

WAKE UP YOUR FACE

First off, you need to know how to keep your skin in good condition, and that means having a good cleansing routine.

1. Start by CLEANING YOUR SKIN. I prefer an oil-free gel. It seems to draw out the dirt from the pores.

2. Smooth toner all over the face with a cotton pad, paying particular attention to the T-zone, cheeks, and neck.

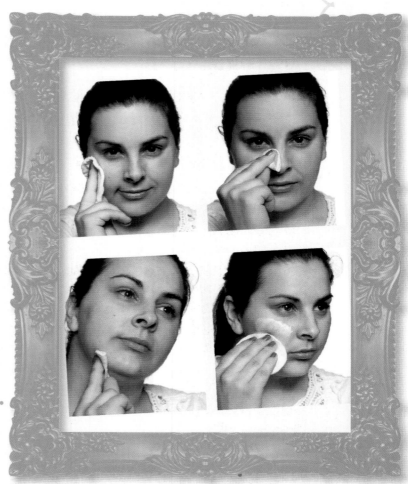

3. Gently massage moisturizer into the face and neck. It can be done by hand, but I prefer to do it with a cotton pad. This replenishes the natural moisture in the skin that the toner has removed.

FLAWLESS FOUNDATION

FOUR STEPS TO FAKING IT

Faces are complicated and not always perfect. There are oily T-zones, spots, blotches, and even different skin tones on different areas of the face. It's the job of primer or moisturizer, concealer, foundation, and finishing powder to iron these out and give a nice, smooth, even look to the face.

I can't recommend specific products because everyone's preference is different, but I can tell you how to pick the best colors for your skin and show you how I created the base for all the looks in this book.

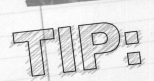

TIP:

THERE IS AN EASY WAY TO CHOOSE THE BEST COLOR FOR CONCEALER AND FOUNDATION. TAKE THREE SHADES THAT ARE LIKELY TO GO WITH YOUR SKIN TONE AND APPLY SIDE BY SIDE ALONG THE JAWBONE. TAKE THE RING FINGER AND SMOOTH EACH ONE INTO THE SKIN. THE COLOR THAT BLENDS INTO YOUR SKIN TONE IS THE ONE TO GO WITH—DISCARD THE OTHERS.

1. Start with a MOISTURIZER or PRIMER. Either product will smooth the skin, make it easier to apply foundation, and help the foundation stay in place.

Apply it all over the face, right up to the hairline. I like to use a cotton pad for this, but you can do it by hand.

2. CONCEALER will cover imperfections and flaws ready for makeup to be applied. It's not for covering the whole face.

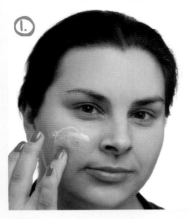

1.

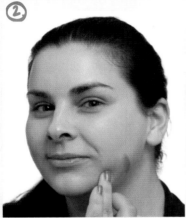

2.

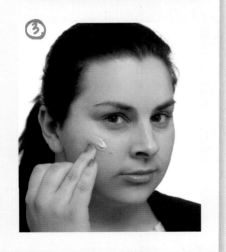

3.

Depending on how you feel about your skin, you can repeat these steps to get a really good finish.

③ FOUNDATION. I use a brush to apply foundation. It's time consuming, but you will get a better effect. If you are in a hurry, there's nothing wrong with using your fingers. Or you can do a bit of both to get into all those nooks and crannies.

BE CAREFUL NOT TO GET FOUNDATION IN YOUR EYES—IT STINGS!

④. FINISHING POWDER. I am starting to learn the value of this extra step—it sets the foundation.

It can either be colored or translucent. To apply, use a really soft fluffy brush to swirl it in a circular motion all over the face and blend well into the foundation.

TIP:

BE SUN SAFE

MOST FOUNDATIONS NOW CONTAIN A SUNSCREEN. IF YOURS DOESN'T, YOU SHOULD THINK ABOUT APPLYING A SUNSCREEN BEFORE THE FOUNDATION. IT'S IMPORTANT TO PROTECT YOUR SKIN. AND YOUR SKIN WILL LOVE THE EXTRA MOISTURIZING LAYER, TOO.

BRONZER, BLUSH, AND HIGHLIGHTER ARE USED TO ENHANCE AND CREATE THE EFFECT OF PERFECT BONE STRUCTURE.

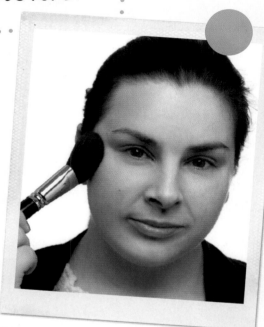

BRONZER

Usually a GOLDEN BROWN BRONZER lends a healthy glow to the skin.

Use a fluffy or kabuki brush to shade the outside area of the face, from the temple, under the cheekbone, and down to the jawline in the **shape of a 3**.

Start off with as little as possible and build it up carefully, to give a glow.

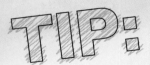

TIP:

TAKE CARE, BECAUSE BRONZER CAN TURN ORANGE ON TOP OF SOME FOUNDATIONS, OR IF YOU PUT TOO MUCH ON. NOT A GOOD LOOK . . .

BLUSH

This brings a flattering rosebud color to the cheeks and brings out the cheekbone. Use a fluffy or kabuki brush again and start with a small amount and build up a little at a time.

Smile to find the apple of your cheek. Gently dab a little color, and sweep it up and down, blending well and moving gradually towards the hairline. This way you won't leave any harsh lines.

CREAM V. POWDER?

It depends on the look you are trying to achieve. I prefer cream to powder because it gives a fresh, dewy look. Powder will give a matte, more airbrushed effect.

You can create many effects with blush, as you will see throughout the book. The Cheryl Cole look, for example, uses two different blush colors.

And you can use bronzer as a blush if you want a golden glow for a beach look. The MEGAN FOX look will show you how.

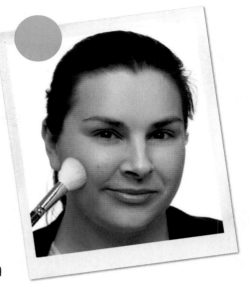

TIP:

SMILE WHEN APPLYING BLUSH. IT NOT ONLY HIGHLIGHTS YOUR CHEEKBONES BUT ALSO CAN LEAD TO A GOOD OLD LAUGH!

HIGHLIGHTER

Highlighter enhances the areas where light would naturally fall, complementing the bone structure. The beautiful shimmery cheeks of the LADY GAGA inspired look will show you how it can work.

Highlighter comes in many shades. Generally, a pale apricot highlighter goes with a bronzed or peach blush, and a pink highlighter complements a pink blush. White or ivory highlighters work with both sets of color. Try them out to see which colors work best with your skin tone.

Use a KABUKI BRUSH to apply the highlighter from the outer eyebrow bone, down along the temple, around and across the top of the cheekbone in a C motion.

YOU CAN ALSO APPLY HIGHLIGHTER FROM THE FOREHEAD, DOWN ALONG THE NOSE, AND ONTO THE CHIN.

FACE FRAMING

EYEBROW-SHAPING SECRETS

EYEBROWS ARE OUR LITTLE FRIENDS, THEY FRAME THE FACE AND WILL SET OFF YOUR LOOK. IN THE CHAPTERS THAT FOLLOW YOU WILL BE ABLE TO SEE HOW EVEN SLIGHTLY DIFFERENT SHAPES CAN DRAMATICALLY ALTER THE OVERALL LOOK.

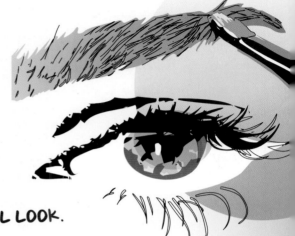

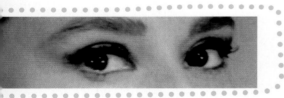

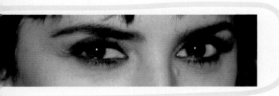

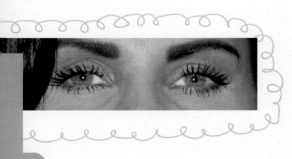

Eyebrows can be SQUARED, ARCHED, ROUNDED, CURVED, or almost straight across. You can see how different my eyebrows can look with Audrey Hepburn's squared look, Penélope Cruz's thick, curved brows, or Katie Price's beautifully rounded eyebrows.

Nobody's eyebrows are identical, so accept that and don't overdo trying to make them look exactly the same.

Different cultures prefer to style their eyebrows in different ways. Sometimes it's to do with fashion as well. Thick, bushy eyebrows can be in one minute, and Moulin Rouge—style pencil-thin eyebrows the next.

When choosing an EYEBROW POWDER, look for something on a par with your natural hair color. Don't go for anything too dark.

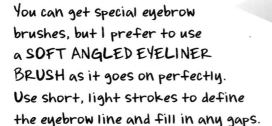

You can get special eyebrow brushes, but I prefer to use a SOFT ANGLED EYELINER BRUSH as it goes on perfectly. Use short, light strokes to define the eyebrow line and fill in any gaps.

If you have healthy eyebrows, use VASELINE instead of wax and powder to spruce up the shape. The glossy finish freshens the face and helps make you look younger.

EYEBROW WAX or gel will help to keep the shape and ensure you don't have stray hairs.

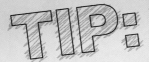

TIP:

NEVER OVERPLUCK— OR YOU WON'T GET TO CHOOSE WHETHER YOU PREFER THICK OR THIN

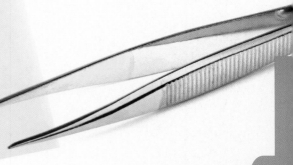

EYE PRIMER

THIS ACTS AS A BASE AND GIVES EYESHADOW INTENSITY. IT REALLY MAKES THE COLORS POP!

There are two different types: one with a matte base and the other with a frosted base. The matte base will give a more powdered finish, and the frosted base will give a metallic effect. Sometimes you need to apply two layers to get a good base, or you can put a little powder of a similar color over a cream base to set it.

My kits all have EYE PRIMER because it's such an important part of the preparation. And remember that it doesn't always have to be white, ivory, or beige in color. In the LEONA LEWIS look I use black primer.

Apply primer all over the eyelid and usually up to the eyebrow in a stroking motion.

Liquid eyeliner can be scary to use! If you are dead confident, apply directly with the applicator. Or you can cheat and use an angled eyeliner brush, which gives you slightly better control.

Eyeliner pencils are easier to use, and there are plenty available that are soft and creamy rather than hard and sharp. They are ideal for using on the tight line and water line.

Rest your little finger on your cheek to help keep your hand steady.

WATER LINE

This is the narrow, wet part just above the lower lash line. You can use a creamy eyeliner pencil here to define and bring out the whites of eyes.

It does tend to come off though, even if you use a waterproof eyeliner pencil. So you will have to keep reapplying at intervals. And check that it hasn't migrated to the inner corner!

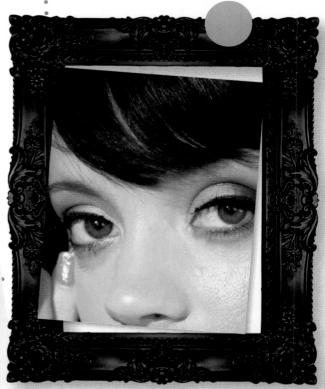

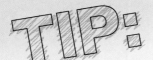

TIP:
NEVER USE LIQUID EYELINER ON THE WATER LINE OR TIGHT LINE. ONLY USE A SOFT, CREAMY EYELINER PENCIL, OR YOU'LL BE CRYING FOR DAYS!

TIGHT LINE

This is great for defining and framing eyes. Once your mascara is on it will give the appearance of thicker lashes. It tickles at first, but you will get used to it—so practice.

Hold your top eyelashes back with your forefinger and gently stroke a creamy eyeliner pencil along the wet part below the lashes. Start at the outer corner and work your way in. This is a very delicate area, so you need a pencil that is as smooth and creamy as possible.

If you are using this technique, it should be a first step, before the eye primer.

TIP:

SOMETHING ELSE I'VE JUST LEARNED—IF YOUR EYES ARE FEELING TIRED OR SORE, PUT TWO SILVER SPOONS IN ICED WATER AND THEN HOLD THEM AGAINST THE EYES FOR A FEW MINUTES. IT'S REALLY REFRESHING AND ANY BAGS OR REDNESS WILL DISAPPEAR!

MASCARA

Tip your head right back to apply mascara so you won't catch the skin with the wand. Give your lashes a nice wiggle with the wand from root to tip. Keep the lashes well separated and take care not to smudge.

IT DOESN'T MATTER HOW MANY SILLY FACES YOU PULL WHILE YOU DO THIS—I PULL LOTS!

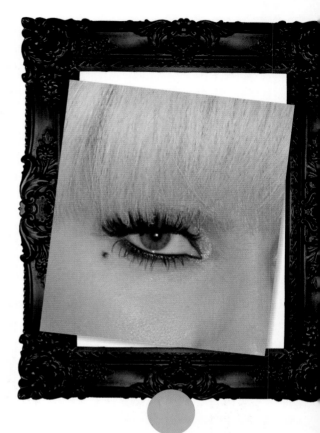

Push the wand upwards for a wide-eyed appearance and sweep it outwards for a sultry, inviting look.

Sometimes you need more than one layer to get the right effect.

Then tilt your head forward to add a touch of mascara on the lower lashes to really frame eyes.

How about thinking of brown mascara for your softer looks? I think you'll be really happy with the outcome.

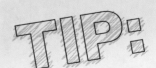

TIP:

I LOVE VIBRANT MASCARA COLORS, TOO. I LIKE TO PUT A COAT OF BLACK MASCARA ON FIRST AND GENTLY TOUCH THE ENDS WITH THE COLOR WAND. IT LOOKS FUNKY, DIFFERENT, AND EXCITING.

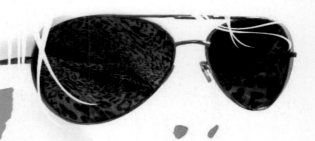

LUSCIOUS LIPS

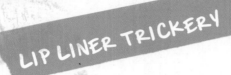

LIP LINER TRICKERY

I TEND TO UNDERPLAY MY LIPS BECAUSE I DON'T THINK THEY ARE ONE OF MY BEST FEATURES. BUT IF THEY ARE ONE OF YOUR FAVORITE ASSETS, THERE ARE LOTS OF DIFFERENT WAYS TO HAVE FUN WITH THEM.

For example, the pout. Matte the lips with powder foundation, take a light-colored lip liner, and draw around the natural line of the lips, bridging the Cupid's bow.

Draw a line on the lower lip very slightly below the natural lip line, but don't go into the corners. This will make the bottom lip look thicker as well.

Then apply a nude lipstick all over the lips and up to the lip line (it should still show through).

Finish with a clear or light shimmery lip gloss applied to the middle of the lower lip only.

Or if you want to create a fuller look for thin lips, use a lip liner to trace just beyond the natural line on the top and bottom lips. Fill in with your chosen lipstick.

Keep your lips in good condition with Vaseline or lip balm. They are a great base for lipstick, giving a more stained effect.

DESERT ISLAND MUST-HAVES

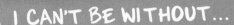

I CAN'T BE WITHOUT...

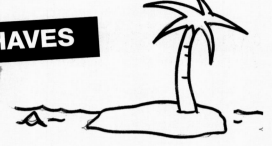

1. **MAC PLUSH LASH MASCARA**—I've tried many mascaras in my time, and none of them quite open your eyes like this one.

2. **L'ORÉAL HIP PURE PIGMENT SHADOW STICKS**—One of the most affordable high-pigment shadows.

3. **KIEHL'S CENTELLA RECOVERY SKIN SALVE**—A moisturizing cream that makes your skin feel as smooth as glass—amazingly soothing after a long day.

4. **MY BLENDER BRUSH**—This dome-shaped brush can do things no other brush can do. Without this brush, I feel like an artist without an arm.

5. **E.L.F. HYPERSHINE LIP GLOSS**—So well priced and an amazing range of colors.

6. **CHRISTIAN DIOR PRO CHEEKS ULTRA-RADIANT BLUSH LIMELIGHT**—Whip your cheeks up into a frenzy with this beautifully light and fluffy pearlescent mousse highlighter—the ultimate for that fresh, dewy look.

7. **STILA CONVERTIBLE EYE PENCIL**—Super creamy pen style, glides smoothly on your skin and water line—gone are the days of the hard, skin-ripping pencil. Onyx is my favorite color.

8. **LANCÔME FLASH RETOUCHE**—It's great for touch-ups on the go—not too creamy, not too matte, just right. And it's got a fab brush applicator to get into all those nooks and crannies.

9. **PAMPERS SENSITIVE WIPES**—If it's good enough for a baby's bottom, it's good enough for my face. Terrific for almost everything—cleaning your face and brushes and clearing up any fallout.

10. **VASELINE**—I always have this at hand. If you don't want to wear makeup but still want to look "alive," put a little on the eyebrows, lips, and lashes.

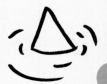

MY FAVORITE BRUSHES

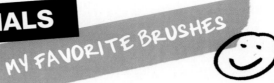

BLENDER BRUSH

My favorite brush. Nice and fluffy with great bristles that create a multitude of effects.

ANGLED EYELINER BRUSH

This has lots of uses—it's great for applying eyeliner along the top and bottom lash lines and also for working on the eyebrows.

EYESHADOW BRUSH

Great for dabbing eyeshadow directly onto the eyelid. It's a good shape, gives controlled application and good coverage.

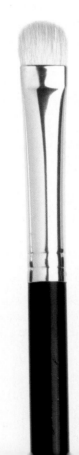

BY LAUREN LUK

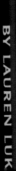

BLUSHER BRUSH

An indespensable, soft-bristle brush that is just the right size for more controlled coverage of blushers and bronzers.

STIPLING BRUSH

Probably the most versatile brush there is. Use to apply liquid foundation, cream blush, powder blush, bronzer, and basically anything you can think of!

SQUARED EYELINER BRUSH

Also very useful— for applying color to the upper and lower lash lines, for creating a smoky effect, and for work on the eyebrows as well.

FOUNDATION BRUSH

I use this every time. There are different sizes— the larger one covers a bigger area and works on the cheeks and jawline, and the smaller one allows more control and works best around the eyes and chin.

FLUFFY BRUSH

This short, flat brush is good for applying blush and bronzer.

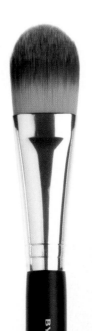
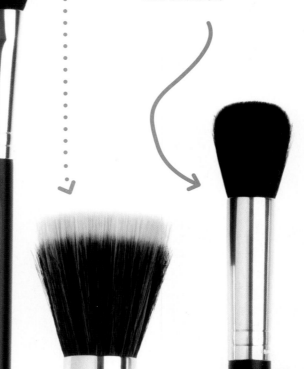
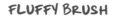

BY LAUREN LUKE

PAINT BOX

HOW TO CHOOSE THE RIGHT COLORS FOR YOU

I AM ALWAYS BEING ASKED WHICH COLORS BEST SUIT PARTICULAR EYE OR HAIR COLORS, SO HERE ARE SOME GENERAL POINTERS THAT I HOPE YOU WILL FIND HELPFUL. DON'T BE AFRAID TO EXPERIMENT THOUGH!

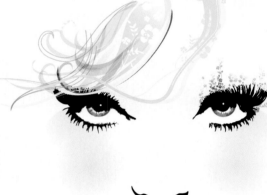

BLOND HAIR AND
GRAY EYES
Dark blue eyeshadow
Mid-pink blush
Nude-peach lips

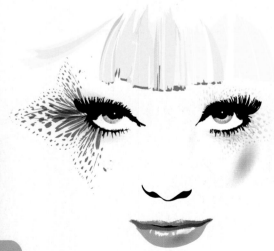

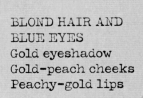

BLOND HAIR AND
BLUE EYES
Gold eyeshadow
Gold-peach cheeks
Peachy-gold lips

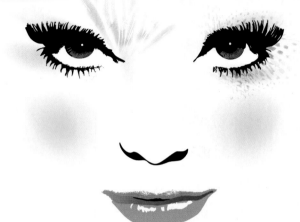

BLOND HAIR AND
BROWN EYES
Lilac eyeshadow
Raspberry blush
Rosy-pink lips

AS YOU GET OLDER...

Your SKIN PIGMENTATION will change, and your HAIR will lighten, so you won't be able to wear the same colors that you used to.

Always go for the lighter shade of your preferred eyeshadow. It will look a lot milder and won't accentuate wrinkles as much as a dark color.

Think along these lines when picking the formula, too. Go for matte or creamy satin and stay away from shimmers—they can be hard on the tautest of skins.

When choosing lipstick, go for a matte lip liner, avoid anything wet and glossy, and choose softer colors.

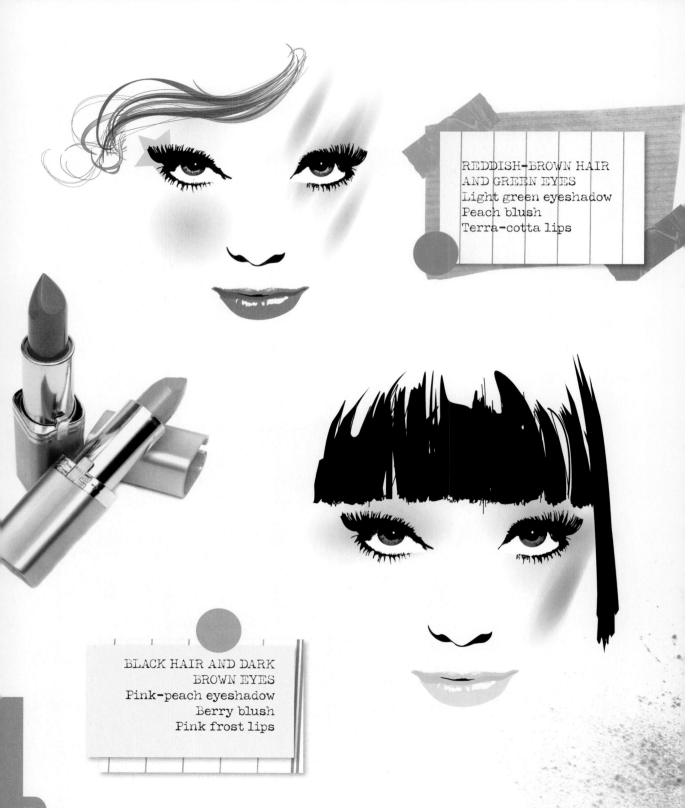

REDDISH-BROWN HAIR
AND GREEN EYES
Light green eyeshadow
Peach blush
Terra-cotta lips

BLACK HAIR AND DARK
BROWN EYES
Pink-peach eyeshadow
Berry blush
Pink frost lips

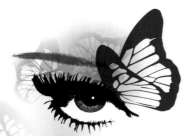
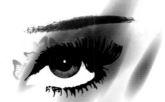
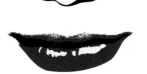

DARK RED HAIR AND
DARK BROWN EYES
Dark green eyeshadow
Terra-cotta blush
Deep cherry lips

COVERING DARK CIRCLES

I LOVE TO USE CONCEALER PENS WHENEVER I HAVE ANY DARKNESS AROUND MY EYES.

LOOK FOR A CONSISTENCY THAT'S NOT TOO CREAMY OR TOO MATTE.

YOU MAY NEED A COUPLE OF APPLICATIONS TO BUILD UP THE COLOR TO MATCH YOUR NATURAL SKIN TONE.

AFTER YOU HAVE USED THE CONCEALER, BLOT WITH A LITTLE FACE POWDER TO SET THE MIXTURE AND DELAY THE INEVITABLE CREASING THAT WILL HAPPEN THROUGH THE DAY.

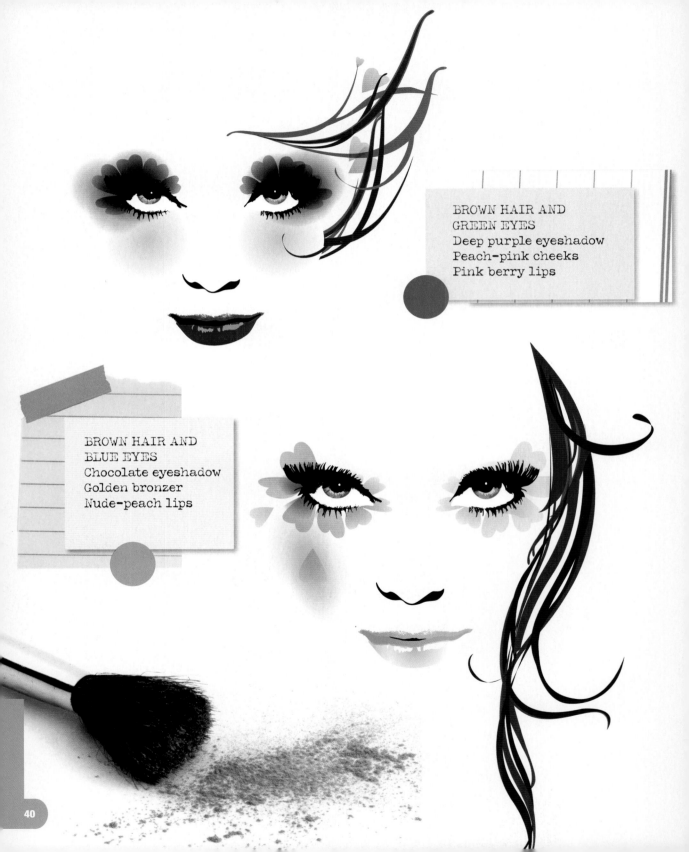

BROWN HAIR AND
GREEN EYES
Deep purple eyeshadow
Peach-pink cheeks
Pink berry lips

BROWN HAIR AND
BLUE EYES
Chocolate eyeshadow
Golden bronzer
Nude-peach lips

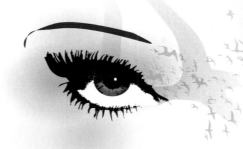

BROWN EYES AND
BROWN HAIR
Green eyeshadow
Peach-bronze cheeks
Dark peach lips

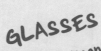

GLASSES

Your eyes are already magnified, so you don't want anything too shimmery. Keep eyeshadow to a matte or slightly satin finish.

You can still wear any color you like, but always make sure you have the lightest color on the majority of the eyelid with the chosen dark or vibrant color added to the crease and just above.

Add a little touch of the stronger color a quarter of the way along the outer lower lash line, too.

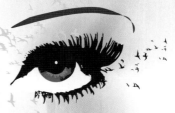

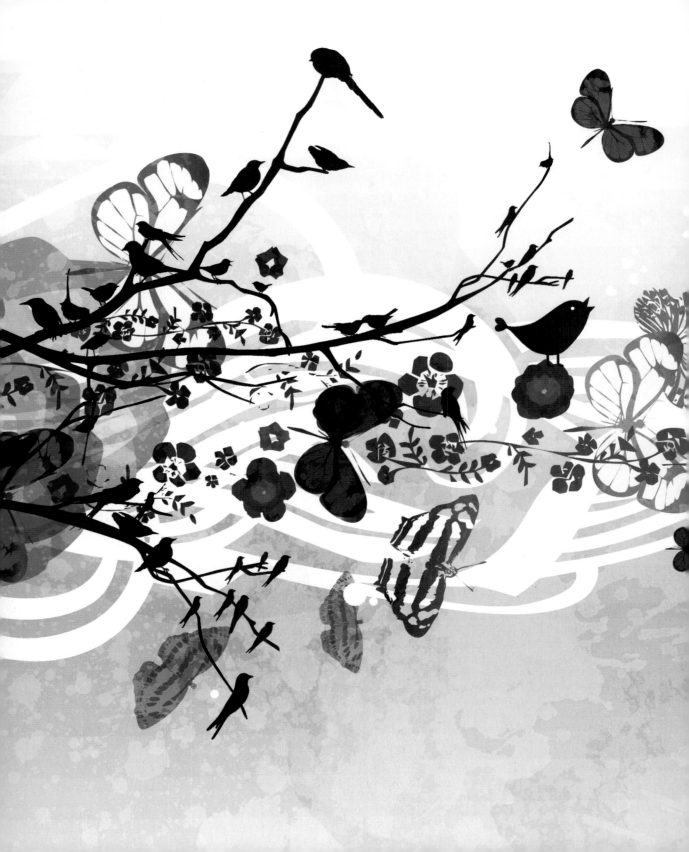

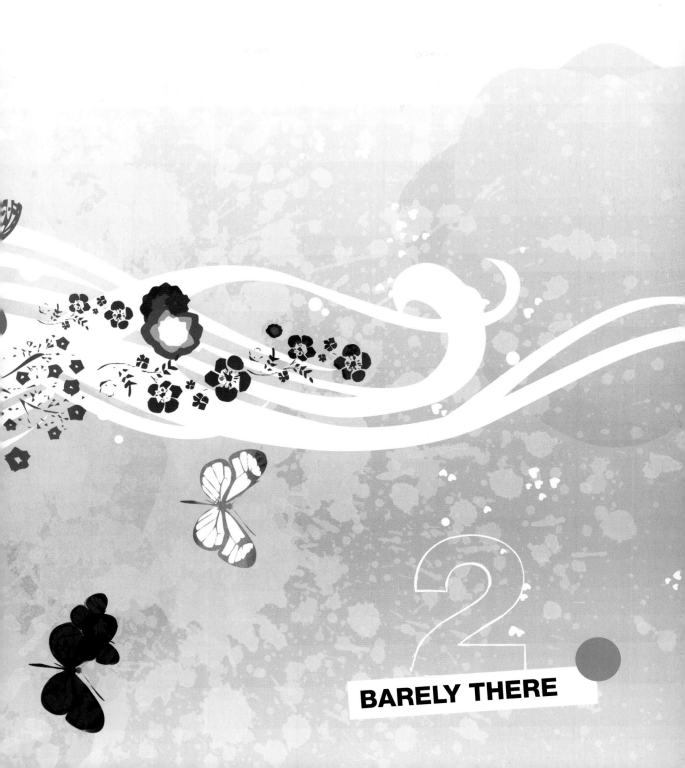

2

BARELY THERE

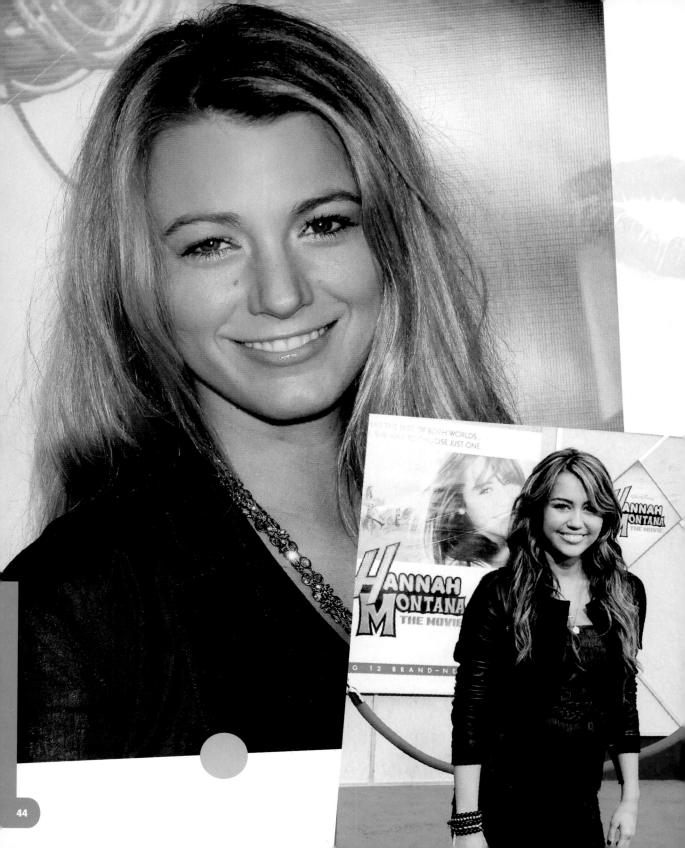

FIRST DATE

BUTTERFLIES AND SECRET KISSES

THIS LOOK, AS SEEN ON BLAKE LIVELY AND MILEY CYRUS, IS SIMPLICITY ITSELF. IT CAN BE DONE IN 5 TO 10 MINUTES, NO PROBLEM, GIVING YOU MORE TIME TO CHECK OUT YOUR OUTFIT.

THE PALETTE

* Ivory creamy eyeshadow
* Silvery-pink frosted eyeshadow
* Black cream eyeliner
* Mid-pink matte powder blush
* Mauve-caffe-latte-colored lipstick
* Peachy-pink lip gloss
* Black mascara

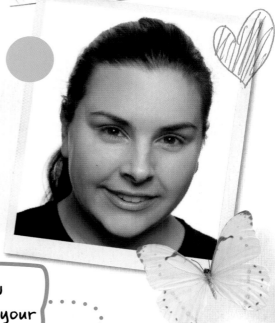

1. Use your third finger to prime the eyelid with an ivory creamy eyeshadow, taking it right up to the eyebrow bone.

Lightly run a little eyeshadow along the lower lash line with your third finger.

Use an eyebrow brush to apply a silvery pink frosted eyeshadow, from the inner corner working across the eyelid in a patting motion and then back and forth across the crease. Extend the color slightly outwards.

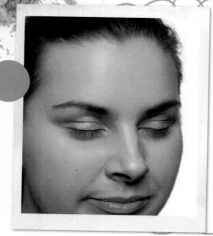

2. Close your eye and, using a creamy black eyeliner pencil, gently tease a light line from halfway across the upper eyelid to the outer edge and just beyond. It should be nice and smoky—but not too much.

3. Dab a fluffy brush into a mid-pink matte powder blush, smile, and apply lightly over the apple of the cheek in an up-down motion, extending almost to the hairline, following the shape of the cheek.

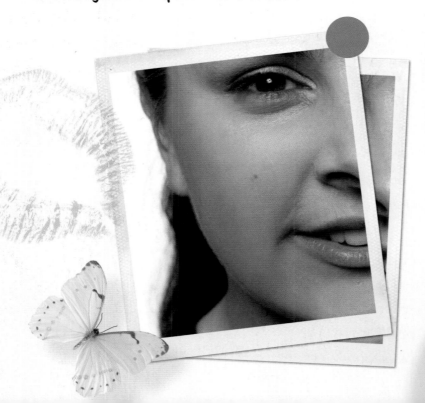

4. THE LIPS. Apply a mauve-caffe-latte-color lipstick, and then a peachy-pink lip gloss. Rub your lips together to blend the colors.

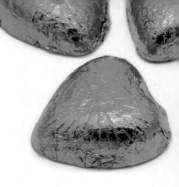

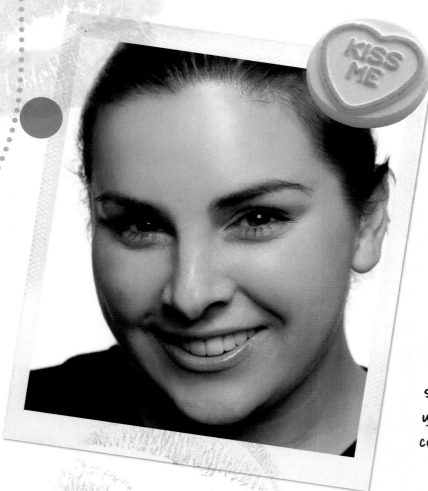

5. MASCARA. Tip your head back and apply a little black mascara to the upper lashes, pushing upwards (not outwards). Be sparing, you don't want your lashes too well covered.

I WANT

TO MAKE ⇒

EVERYONE

FEEL
SPECIAL

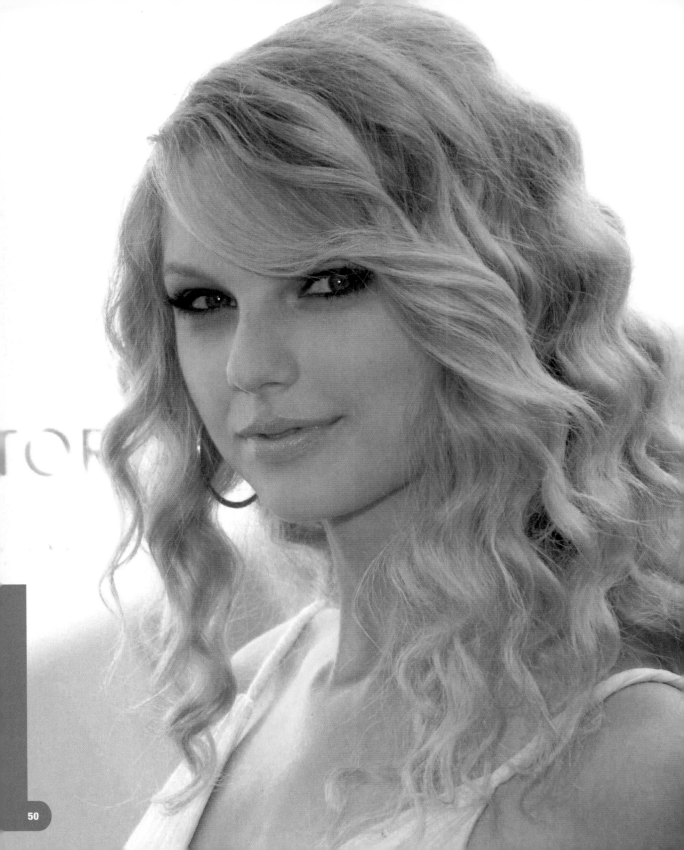

TAYLOR SWIFT

NATURAL GLOW

THIS IS A VERY PRETTY NEUTRAL LOOK, WITH A DASH OF WARMTH IN THE COLORS.

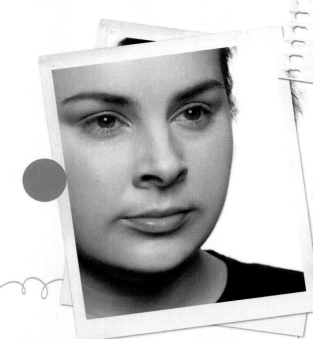

THE PALETTE

* Beige creamy eyeshadow
* Peachy-gold frosted eyeshadow
* White frosted eyeshadow
* Silver-pewter frosted eyeshadow
* Pale peachy-pink frosted blush
* Pearlescent cream highlighter
* Peachy-gold frosted lipstick
* Black mascara

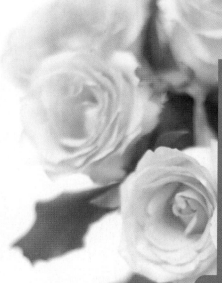

1. With your third finger, prime the eyelid with a BEIGE CREAMY EYESHADOW, going right up to the eyebrow.

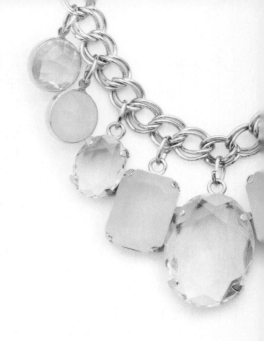

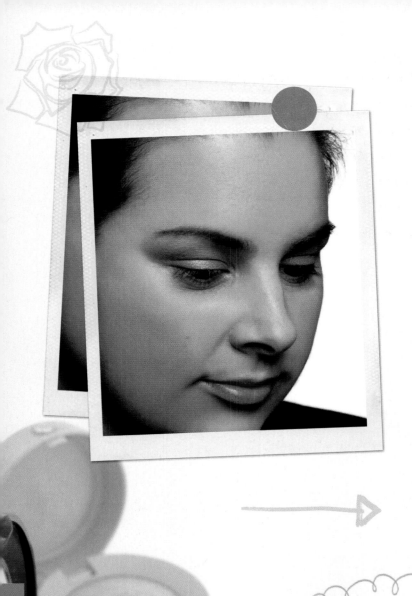

Using an eyeshadow brush, apply a peachy gold frosted eyeshadow all over the eyelid, into the crease, and slightly beyond the outer corner.

Add a tiny bit of WHITE HIGHLIGHTER underneath the eyebrow with your finger, teasing it into the skin, working down to the crease.

② Tilt your head back and, using a blender brush, apply a SILVER-PEWTER FROSTED EYESHADOW. Start from just above the outer crease and gently, in a circular motion, work the color along the crease towards the inner eye, lessening the color as you go. Blend well so it is not too dark.

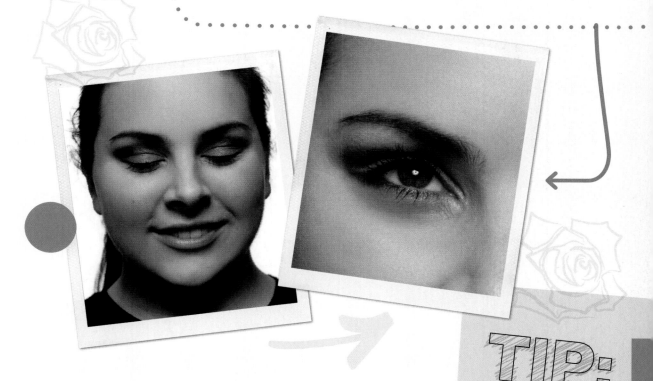

Use an angled eyeliner brush to gently apply the same color under the lower lash line. Work from the middle to the outer corner, feathering as you go, to join the color at the outer corner. Then, with a light touch, take the line two-thirds of the way towards the inner corner.

TIP:

TRY NOT TO GET EYESHADOW IN YOUR EYE —IT HURTS!

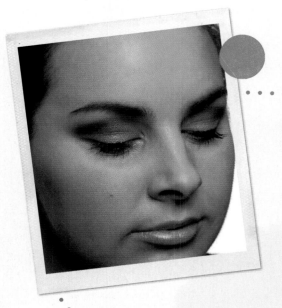

3. Blush and highlighter. Using a fluffy brush, apply a pale peachy-pink frosted blush in a circular motion on the lower apple of the cheek, bringing it out and up to the hairline. BLEND IN WELL.

Using your little finger, dab a tiny bit of pearlescent cream highlighter onto the top part of the cheekbone, out beyond the corner of the eye, and up in a C shape. Blend well.

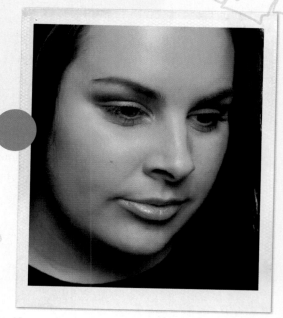

4. With your finger or foundation brush, apply a little foundation to the lips to hold the color and give a neutral base (especially if you have dark lips). Then apply a peachy-gold frosted lipstick.

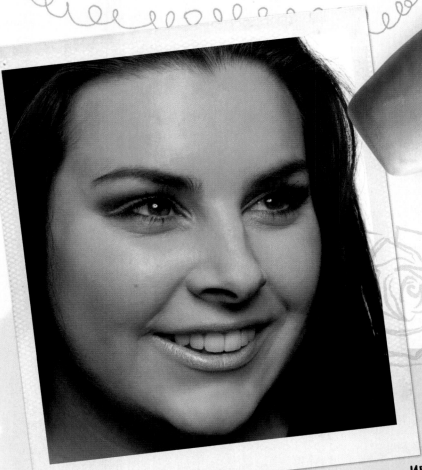

Tilt your head back and apply black mascara in an upwards and outwards motion to the upper lashes. The lower lashes are optional, but I like to do them because it frames your eyes.

SWEET AND INNOCENT BRIDE

HE CAN'T TAKE HIS EYES OFF YOU

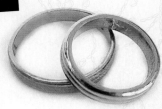

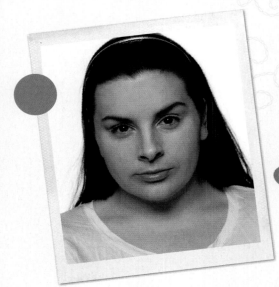

IT'S FRESH AND DEWY CHEEKED, BUT YOU ALSO WANT YOUR GROOM'S HEAD TO TURN. EVEN THOUGH THERE IS NO EYELINER, THIS LOOK HAS BOTH SIMPLICITY AND DEPTH.

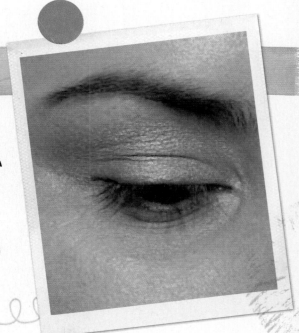

(1.) Prime the eyelid all over to just above the crease with an ivory frosted primer.

Using an eyeshadow brush, apply the pale lilac eyeshadow over the top of the primer.

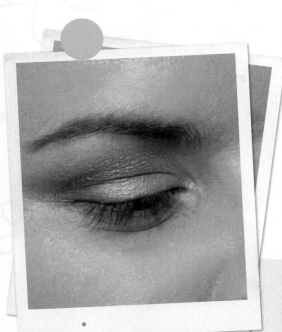

THE PALETTE

* Ivory frosted primer
* Pale lilac frosted eyeshadow
* Grape-colored frosted eyeshadow
* Raspberry matte powder blush
* Cream highlighter
* Matte peach lip liner
* Rosy-gold creamy lipstick
* Black mascara

② Use a blender brush to apply the grape-colored eyeshadow. Dab it onto the outer corner going out to the bone and work back along the crease, pushing the brush into the INNER CORNER.

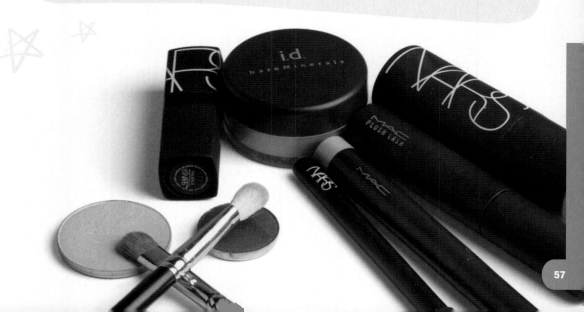

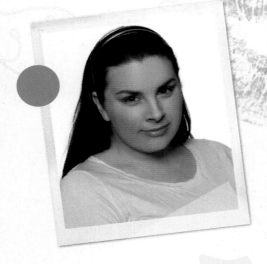

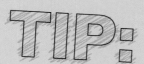

3. Smile, and use a fluffy brush to gently tease the raspberry powder onto the apple of the cheek. Flick the brush back and forth to blend well.

Then apply highlighting cream, starting from the outer eyebrow, down under the eye in the shape of a C, across to the center of the cheekbone. Blend the highlighter into the blush to create the dewy effect.

TIP:

THE DEWY EFFECT IS CREATED BY A COMBINATION OF RASPBERRY MATTE POWDER BLUSH AND A CREAM HIGHLIGHTER.

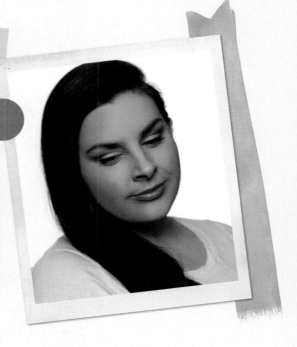

4. THE LIPS. Start by drawing a Cupid's bow with a matte peach lip liner. Make sure it is a good natural color so the line won't look harsh. Outline the top and bottom lips and then fill in with the pencil (you will need something underneath the lipstick when you kiss the groom).

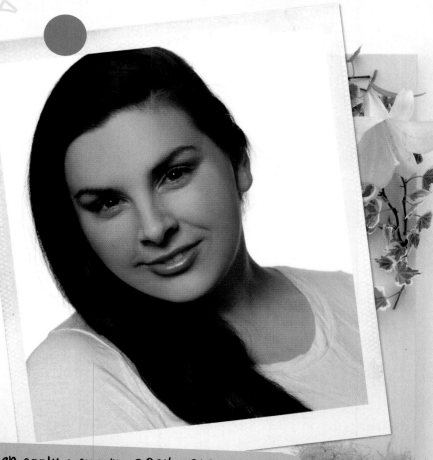

Then apply a creamy ROSY-GOLD LIPSTICK.

Finish with a touch of black mascara—to the top eyelashes only.

OFFICE CHIC
UNDERSTATED AND SO EASY 😊

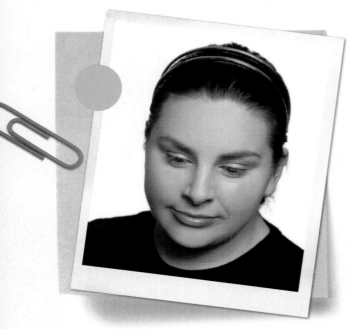

THIS IS A **QUICK LOOK** USING NEUTRAL COLORS WITH LIGHT GOLD AND BROWN. UNDERSTATED FOR WHEN YOU ARE AT WORK, AND PERFECT FOR WHEN YOU ARE IN A HURRY.

1. Use your third finger to apply the primer all over the eyelid to just above the bone.

Use an eyeshadow brush to apply a honey-colored frosted eyeshadow in an up-and-down motion over the eyelid, and then back and forth across the crease. Take the color to the outer edge.

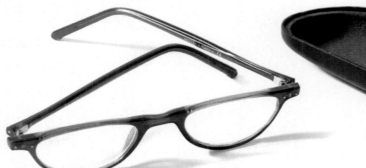

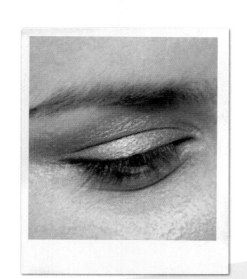

2. Then, using a CHOCOLATE-BROWN eyeliner pencil, draw a fine line along the outer third of the eyelid, close to the lashes, lifting slightly at the corner. Don't blink!

Repeat on the outer third of the bottom lashes, making the line slightly thicker at the corner, and fill in.

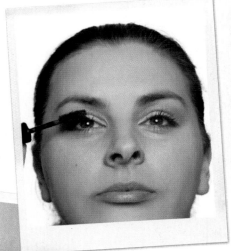

3. Tilt your head back and apply brown mascara to the upper lashes. Add a very light touch to the lower lashes if you like.

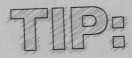

TIP:

BROWN MASCARA IS
BETTER THAN BLACK FOR
THIS LOOK—IT'S SOFTER
AND BLENDS IN WELL WITH
THESE COLORS.

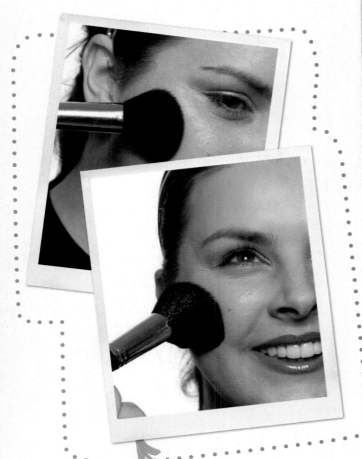

4. Smile, and use a fluffy brush to apply a pale PEACH FROSTED BLUSH on the apple of your cheek. Bring the color right up to the hairline, and blend well.

Now create a CUPID'S BOW. Rest your little finger on your chin and, using a matte coffee lip pencil, outline the inner half of both sides, emphasising slightly the Cupid's bow. Fade the line towards the outer corners.

Then move the pencil back and forth in the center half of the bottom lip, and extend the line to the sides.

TAKE A LIGHT COFFEE-COLORED LIP GLOSS
AND FILL IN THE TOP AND BOTTOM LIPS. BLEND
THE LIP GLOSS WITH THE LIP LINER SO THE
LINE ISN'T OBVIOUS.

January

5 MONDAY

(5-360)

 DO SOMETHING
DIFFERENT EV
DON'T ALLOW
SLIP INTO TH
MAKEUP RUT!

LITTLE

RY DAY SO YOU

URSELF TO

T AWFUL

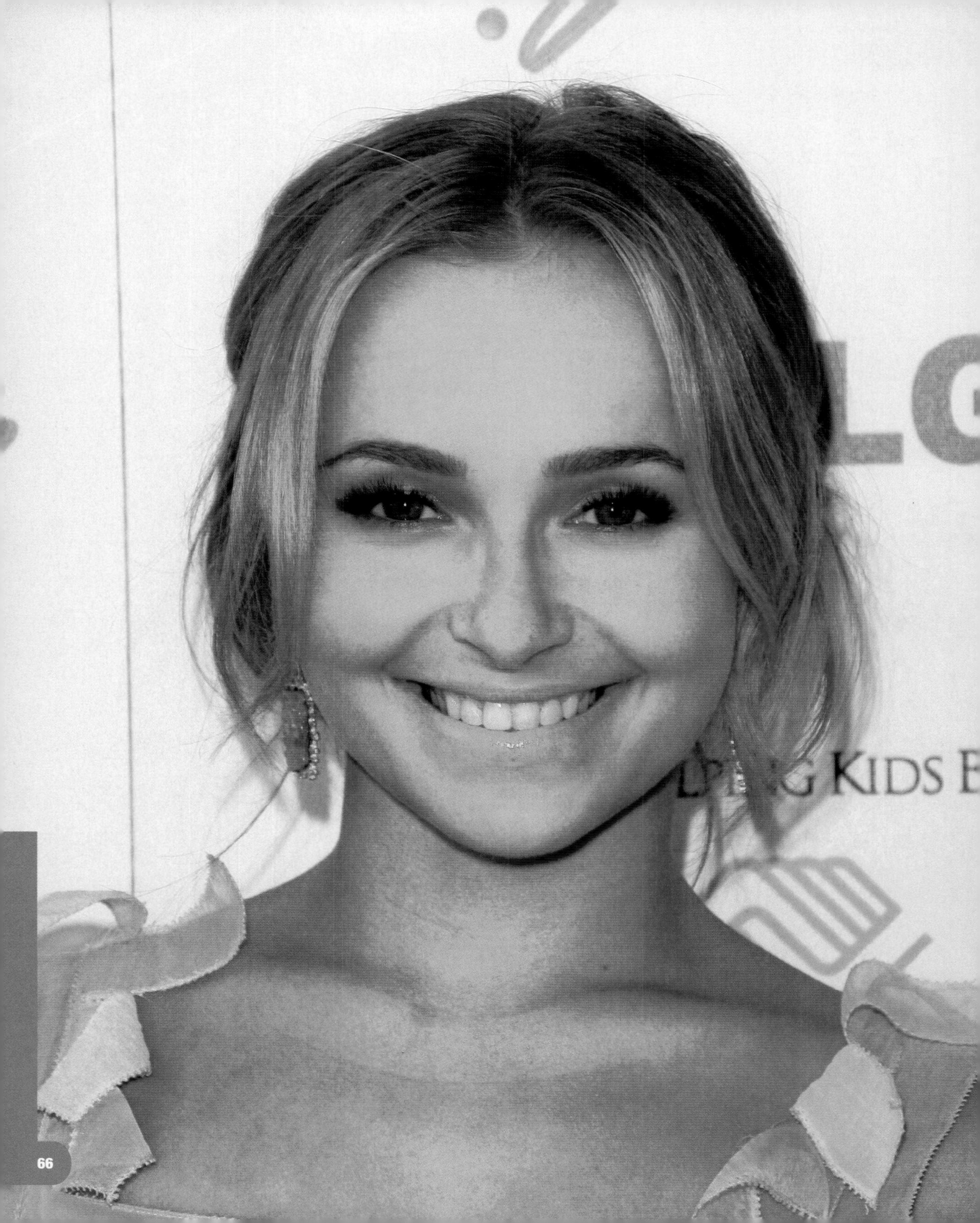
LG
KIDS

HAYDEN PANETTIERE

AMERICAN BEAUTY

A SOFT, SMOKY BUT FRESH LOOK THAT USES GRAY AND BLUE EYESHADOW AND HIGHLIGHTER.

THE PALETTE

* Gray frosted eye mousse
* Light gray-blue frosted eyeshadow
* Medium blue frosted eyeshadow
* Black creamy eyeliner pencil
* Black mascara
* Peachy-gold frosted blush
* Pearlescent highlighter
* Plum lip liner
* Light plum-pink satin lipstick
* Light pink lip gloss

1. To get the smoky base, start by applying a frosted gray eye mousse with your third finger, all over the eyelid and just above the crease, extending slightly at the outer corner.

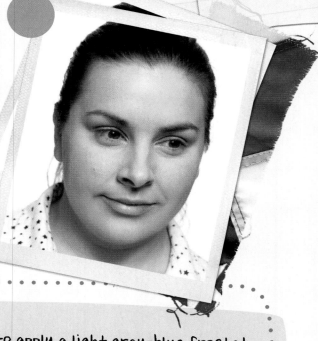

Use an eyeshadow brush to apply a light gray-blue frosted eyeshadow from the inner eye, along the side of the nose and up to meet the gray. Be sparing—it is a subtle highlight to complement the gray.

67

If you would like a little extra highlight, bring the gray-blue outwards above the crease on top of the gray.

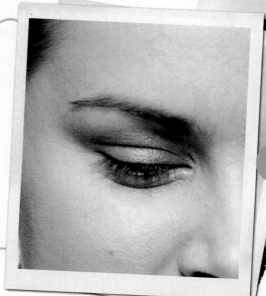

2. Use an eyeshadow brush to gently dab a medium blue frosted eyeshadow on the outer corner only, going a quarter of the way into the crease. Blend well.

Gently lift the eyelid and use a creamy black eyeliner pencil to tight line all the way along the upper eyelid (see page 30).

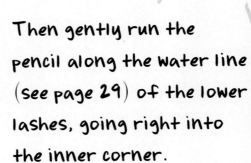

Then gently run the pencil along the water line (see page 29) of the lower lashes, going right into the inner corner.

③ Use the eyeliner pencil to darken the lash line on the upper eyelid at the outer corner only.

Apply black mascara in an upwards motion—you want the eyes to look really awake.

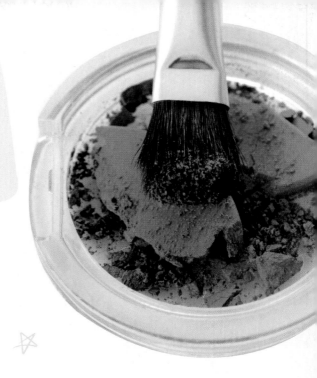

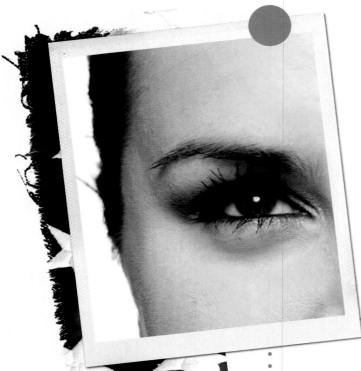

TIP:

BLUE COLOR IMMEDIATELY MAKES THE WHITES OF YOUR EYES BRIGHTER.

Apply a little mascara on the bottom lashes with the tip of the brush.

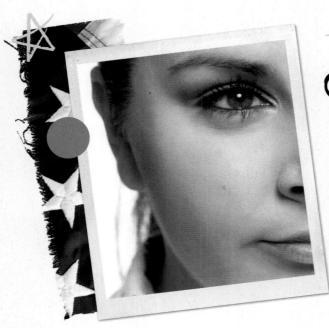

4. Use a kabuki brush to apply the peachy-gold blush under the cheekbone, up towards the hairline. Blend in a circular motion, concentrating under the cheekbone.

Smile, and gently dab a little of the pearlescent highlighter on the top half of the cheekbone and smooth into the skin.

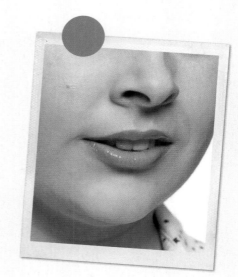

Then dab a little of the highlighter along the middle of the nose, and blend in well.

5. Use a plum lip liner to trace the lip line, then fill in with a light plum-pink satin lipstick.

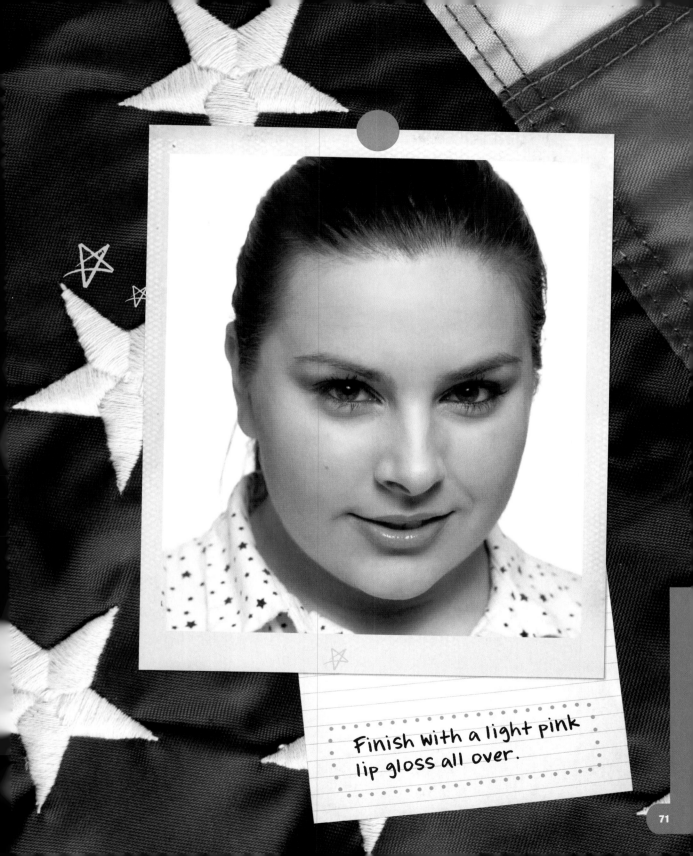

Finish with a light pink lip gloss all over.

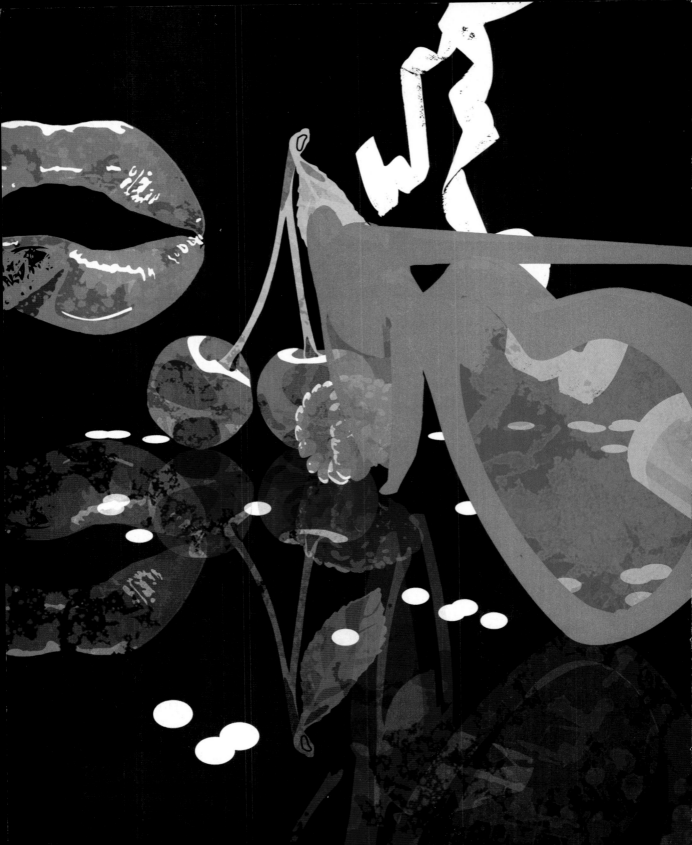

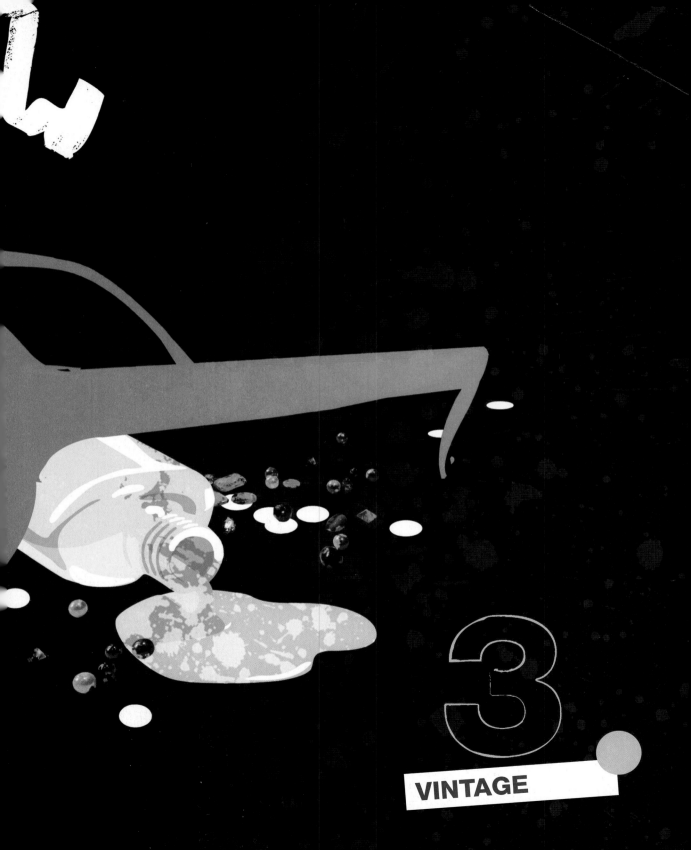

VINTAGE

3.

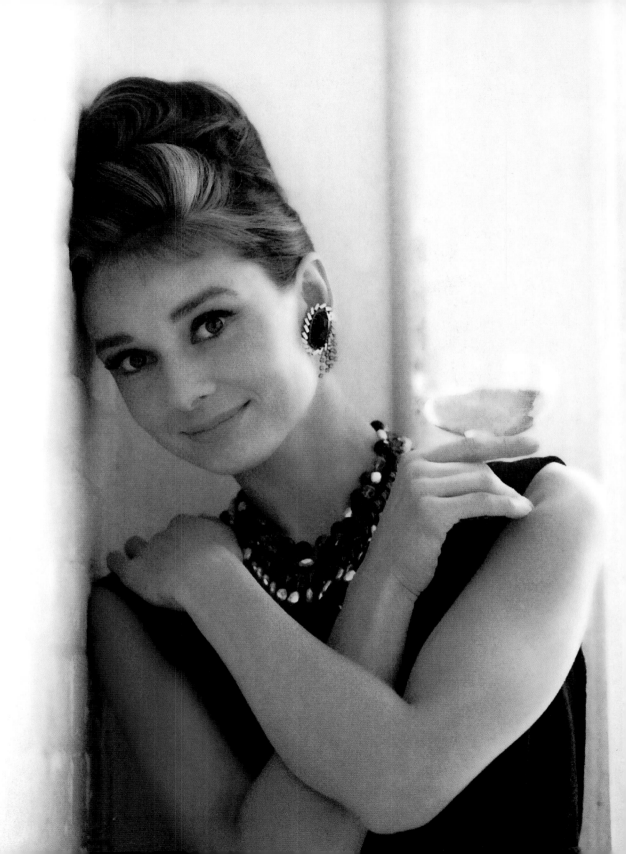

AUDREY HEPBURN

THE EYES HAVE IT

WHEN I THINK OF **AUDREY HEPBURN,** I THINK OF STRONG EYEBROWS AND SOFT LIPS. THIS LOOK USES A LOT OF EYELINER, TOO—ALL THE WAY ACROSS THE EYELID WITH A CUTE FLICK AT THE END.

THE PALETTE

* Mid-gray frosted cream eyeshadow
* Black cream eyeliner
* Dark mauve-plum matte blush
* Mid-pink lipstick with a satin finish
* Eyebrow gel
* Dark brown eyebrow powder
* Black mascara

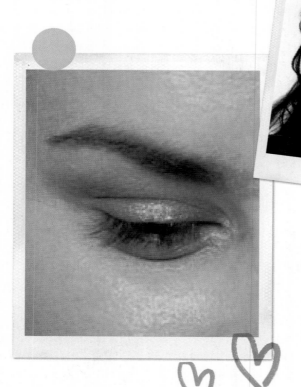

1. Using your ring finger, prime the eyelid with a mid-gray frosted eyeshadow, going a little above the crease at the outside edge.

2. Take an angled eyeliner brush to apply the black eyeliner. Hold your eyelid steady. Start at the very inner corner and gently feather a line as close as possible to the lashes towards the outer corner. The line should be thicker on the inner half so that when you look straight ahead, you don't see any of the eyelid on the inner half—only the black line.

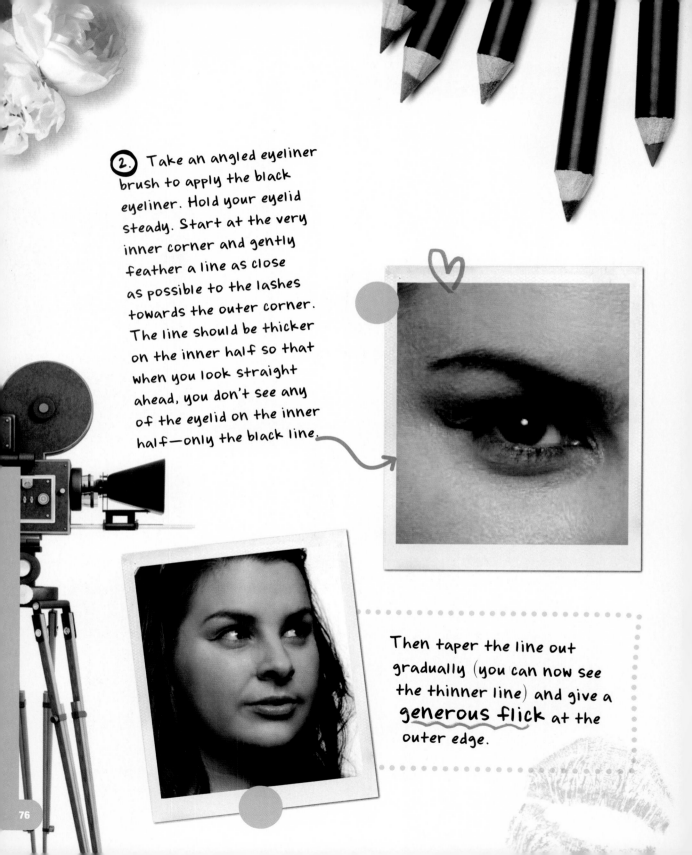

Then taper the line out gradually (you can now see the thinner line) and give a **generous flick** at the outer edge.

3. Using a fluffy brush, apply the dark mauve-plum matte blush, drawing a straight line from the hairline to slightly below the apple of the cheek.

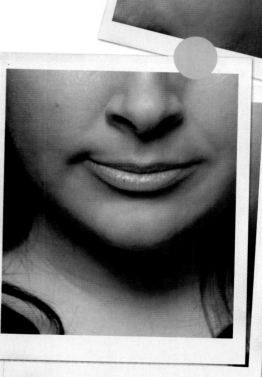

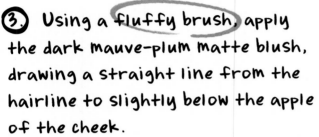

THE LIPS SHOULD LOOK NATURAL. You will need to moisturize before applying a mid-pink lipstick with a satin finish.

4. EYEBROWS. Moisten a square eyeliner brush with a little clear brow gel. Start on the inner corner and gently push the brows up until you reach the arch. Then use the same brush to apply the dark brown eyebrow powder and fill out the underneath of the brow (removing most of the arch) to create a squared effect.

TIP:

You need a lot of mascara. Apply up and outwards (towards the end of your eyebrow), paying more attention to the outer lashes. You will need two to three layers.

FINISH WITH A LIGHT TOUCH OF MASCARA ON THE LOWER LASHES.

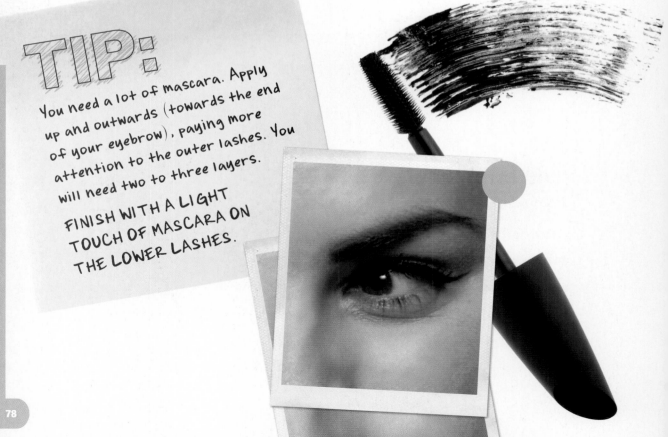

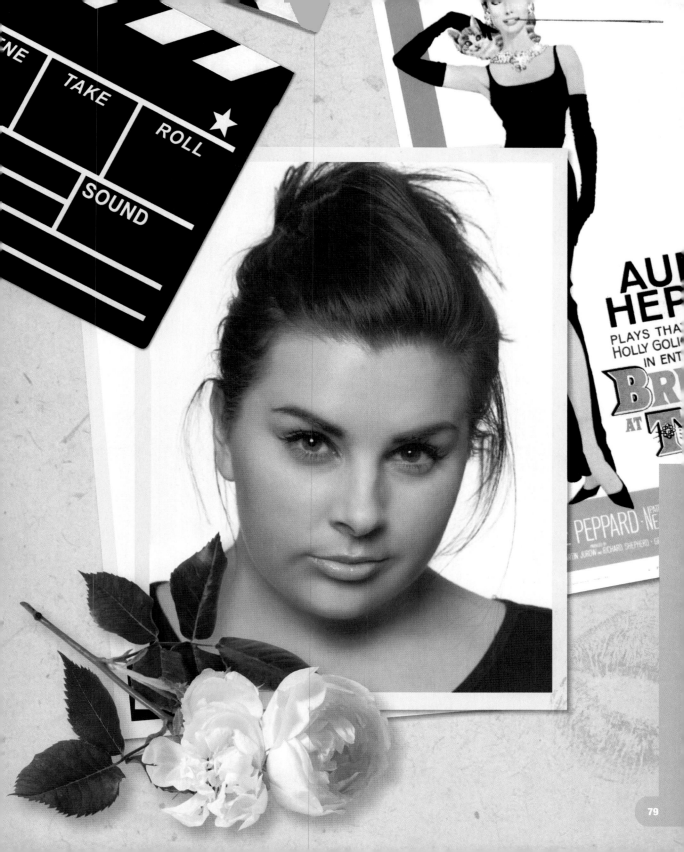

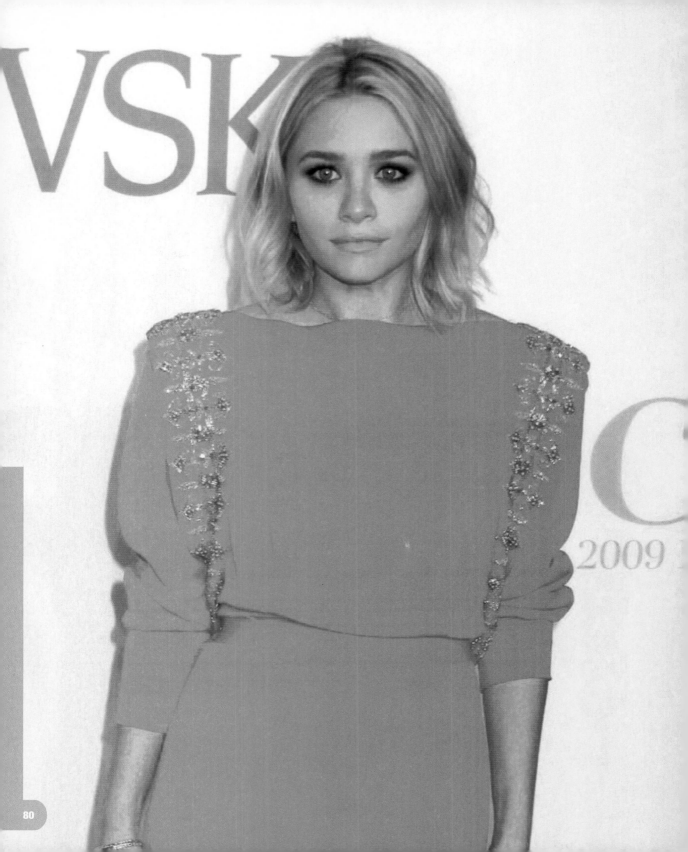

ASHLEY OLSEN

HIPPIE CHICK

A CHOCOLATE-BROWN, SMOKY LOOK—BEAUTIFULLY DEWY BUT WITH A SULTRY DARK SMUDGING UNDER THE EYES.

THE PALETTE

* Eyebrow wax
* Dark brown eyebrow powder
* Golden brown frosted eyeshadow
* Dirty gold eyeshadow
* Black eyeliner pencil
* Black mascara
* Peachy-pink frosted blush
* Ivory pearlescent highlighter
* Powder foundation
* Pale lilac-pink matte lipstick

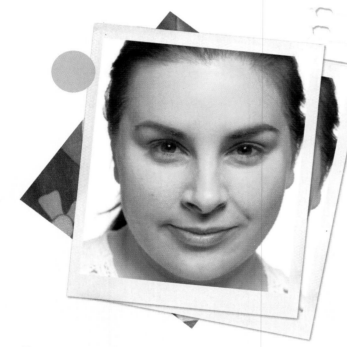

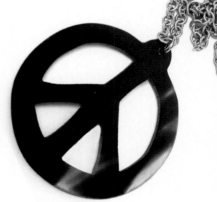

1. The first step is the eyebrows. THE LOOK IS QUITE SQUARED. Use a squared eyeliner brush to apply eyebrow wax along the brow. Then apply a dark brown eyebrow powder all over the brow, teasing the color to get the squared effect.

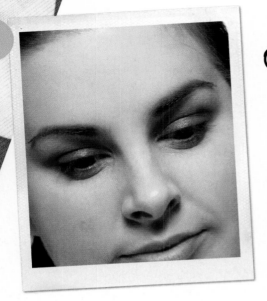

2. Using a blender brush, apply a golden brown frosted eyeshadow gently across the upper eyelid, paying more attention to the lash line and taking the color straight across the eyelid in a rectangular shape. Blend well into the lash line.

Use the same brush to cover the brown eyeshadow with a dirty gold eyeshadow to give a bit of a shimmer.

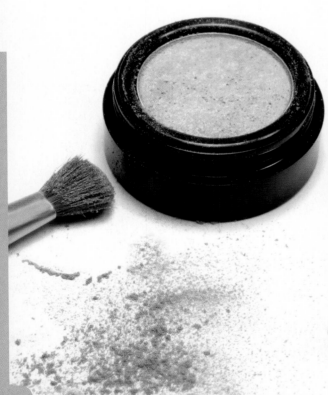

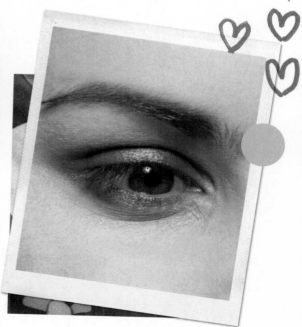

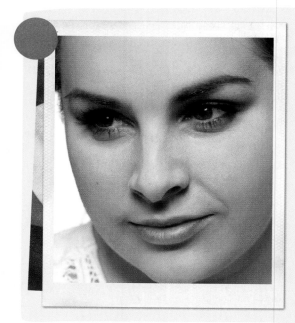

Take an angled eyeliner brush and apply the brown and then the gold eyeshadow all the way along the lower lash line. Blend well.

③ Using a black creamy eyeliner pencil, draw a fine line along the outer quarter of the upper eyelid as close to the lashes as possible to just beyond the outer corner.

Repeat on the lower lash line, and smudge the color with a sponge-tipped brush.

Apply black mascara, wiggling the brush as you go to get the lashes well separated and as long as you can get them. Use an UPWARDS MOTION and keep applying until you are happy. I applied three layers.

ADD A TOUCH OF MASCARA TO THE LOWER LASHES.

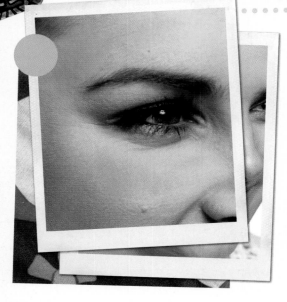

Use a kabuki brush to apply a peachy pink blush all over the cheekbone in a circular motion.

4. Dust the lips with a powder foundation and finish with a pale lilac-pink matte lipstick.

Use the same brush to apply the ivory PEARLESCENT HIGHLIGHTER over the top. Add a touch along the nose.

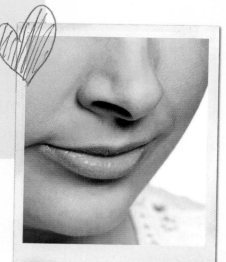

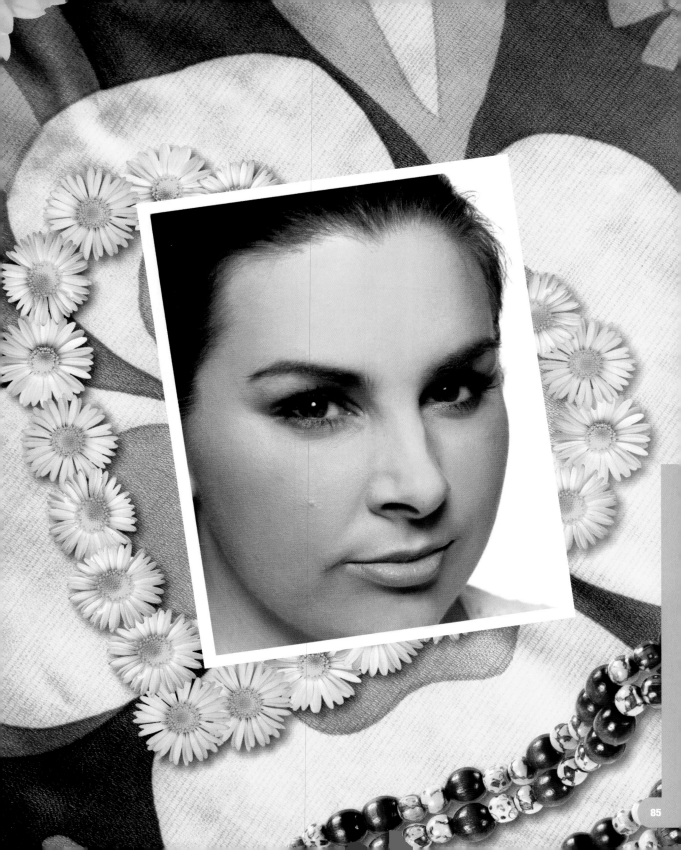

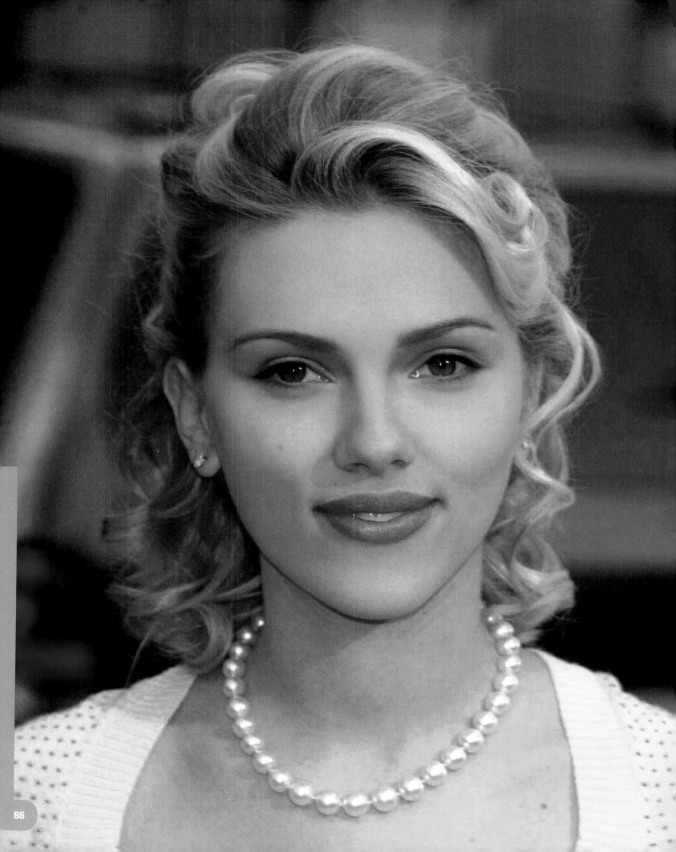

1950S BABY DOLL
THE WOW FACTOR

THIS **LOOK**, WORN STRIKINGLY BY SCARLETT JOHANSSON, IS INSPIRED BY 1950S AMERICAN ADVERTISEMENTS. IT'S **FUN**, IT'S COLORFUL, AND IT'S SLIGHTLY KITSCH!

THE PALETTE

* Cream frosted eyeshadow
* Matte cream eyeshadow
* Black liquid eyeliner
* Bright red lip liner
* Bright red lipstick
* Black mascara
* Eyebrow gel
* Dark brown eyebrow shader
* Dark dolly-pink blush
* Black eyeliner pencil

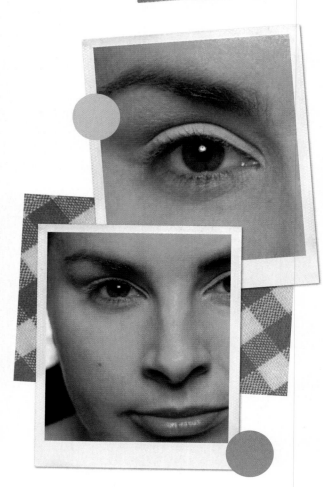

1. Use your third finger to prime the eye with a cream frosted eyeshadow, all the way up to the eyebrow. And then with your little finger, run the color under the eye to light the whole eye area.

Again with your third finger, apply the matte cream eyeshadow over the top of the primer on the eyelid and just past the crease.

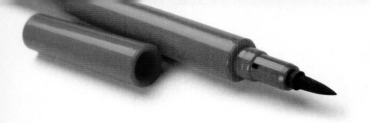

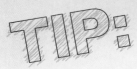

TIP:

ALWAYS, ALWAYS TAKE YOUR MAKEUP OFF BEFORE BED BECAUSE IF YOU THINK YOUR SKIN IS BAD NOW, JUST WAIT TILL THE MORNING... IT'S SO IMPORTANT TO ALLOW YOUR SKIN TO BREATHE THROUGH THE NIGHT.

2. Use an angled eyeliner brush to apply black liquid eyeliner—we want a THICK BLACK LINE. Rest the little finger on your cheek and, starting in the middle of the upper eyelid, draw a line extending to the outer edge and finishing with a small flick. Then, from the inner corner, make a line to meet in the middle—the line should look rounded all the way along.

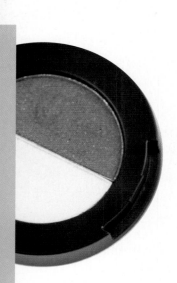

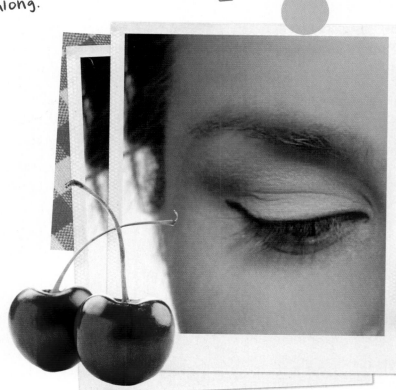

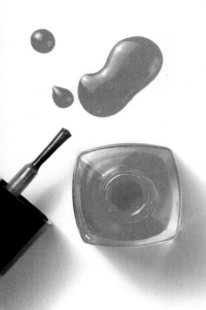

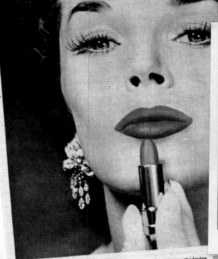

Don't dye your lips. Don't dry your lips. Give your lips the lustre, the loving care of Max Factor Color-Fast Lipstick.

Twelve glamorous, glowing shades . . . with lustre that lasts the live-long day. With lanolin too, to keep your lips so soft, so smooth. No other lipstick takes such loving care of your lips. No other lipstick keeps your lips so excitingly kissable. Now you can give your lips the loveliness you long for. Use Max Factor Color-Fast Lipstick—most-wanted lipstick

COLOR-F

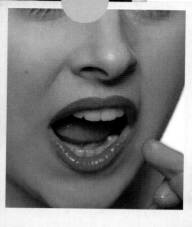

In golden swivel-cases only
5/- Refills **2/9**

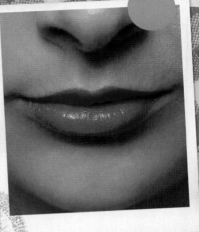

(3.) For **red, red lips**, use a bright red lip liner and draw a line slightly beyond the natural line on the top and bottom lips. Fill in with a bright red lipstick.

BE BRAVE—
YOU'LL LOOK
FANTASTIC!

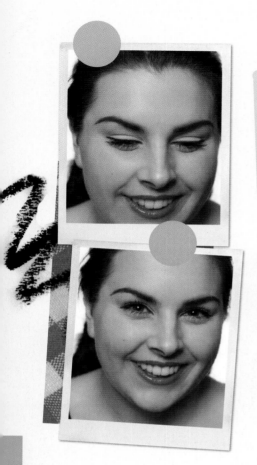

Apply mascara to the upper lashes only, upwards and outwards (towards the end of your eyebrow), being careful to draw out and emphasize the outer lashes.

The eyebrows need to be **emphasized**. Dab a square eyeliner brush into an eyebrow gel or a wet wipe. Use a dark brown eyebrow powder to **enhance** your natural line and create a rounded (not arched) eyebrow.

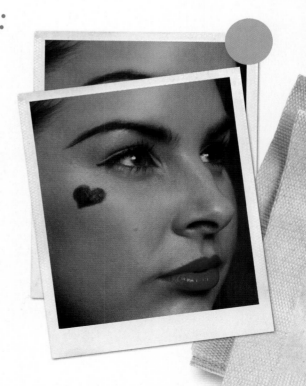

4. Use a brush to apply a dark dolly-pink blush. Smile and blend well in a circular motion onto the apple of the cheek.

Now for the **fun** part—use a black eyeliner pencil to draw a small heart on your cheek.

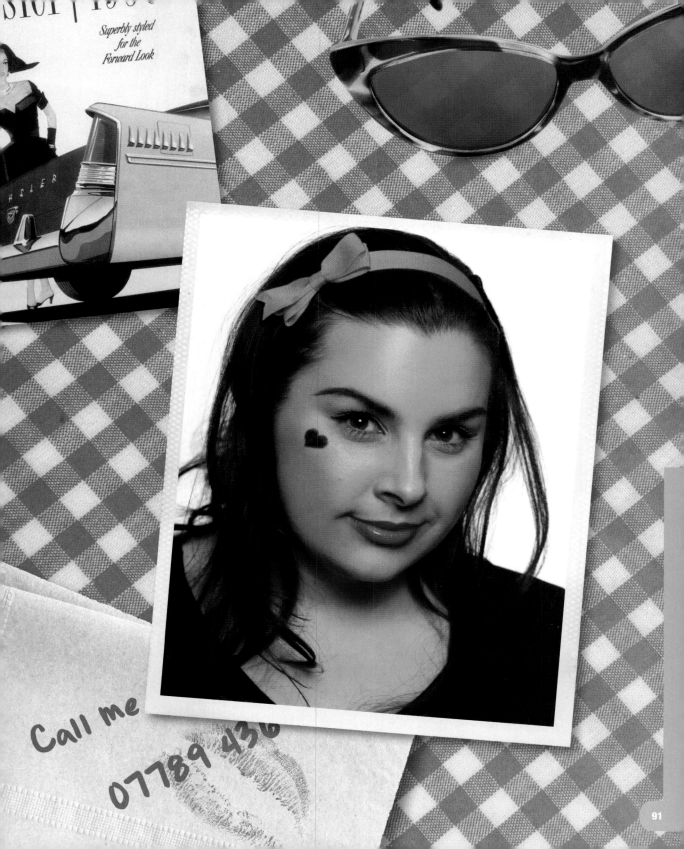

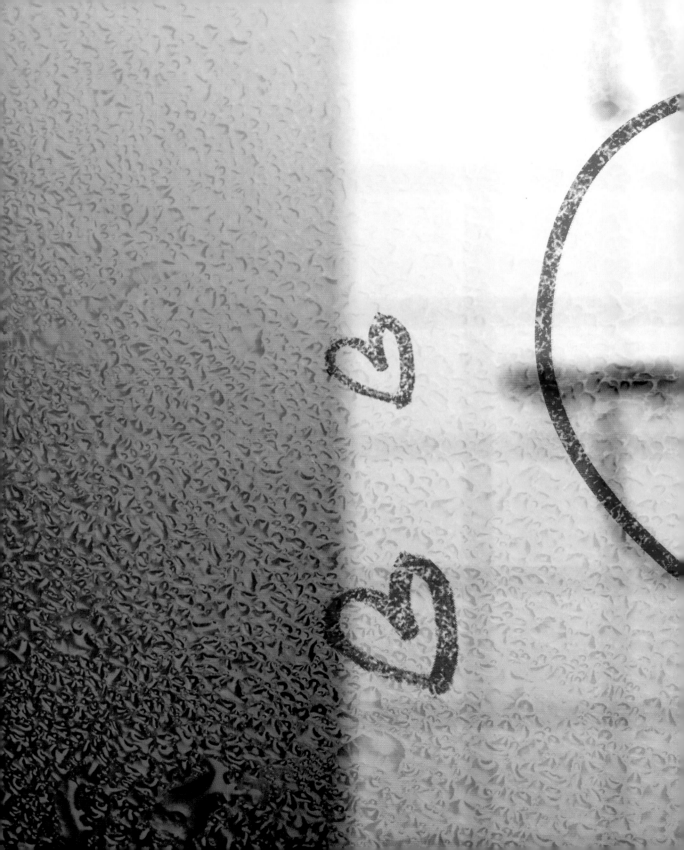

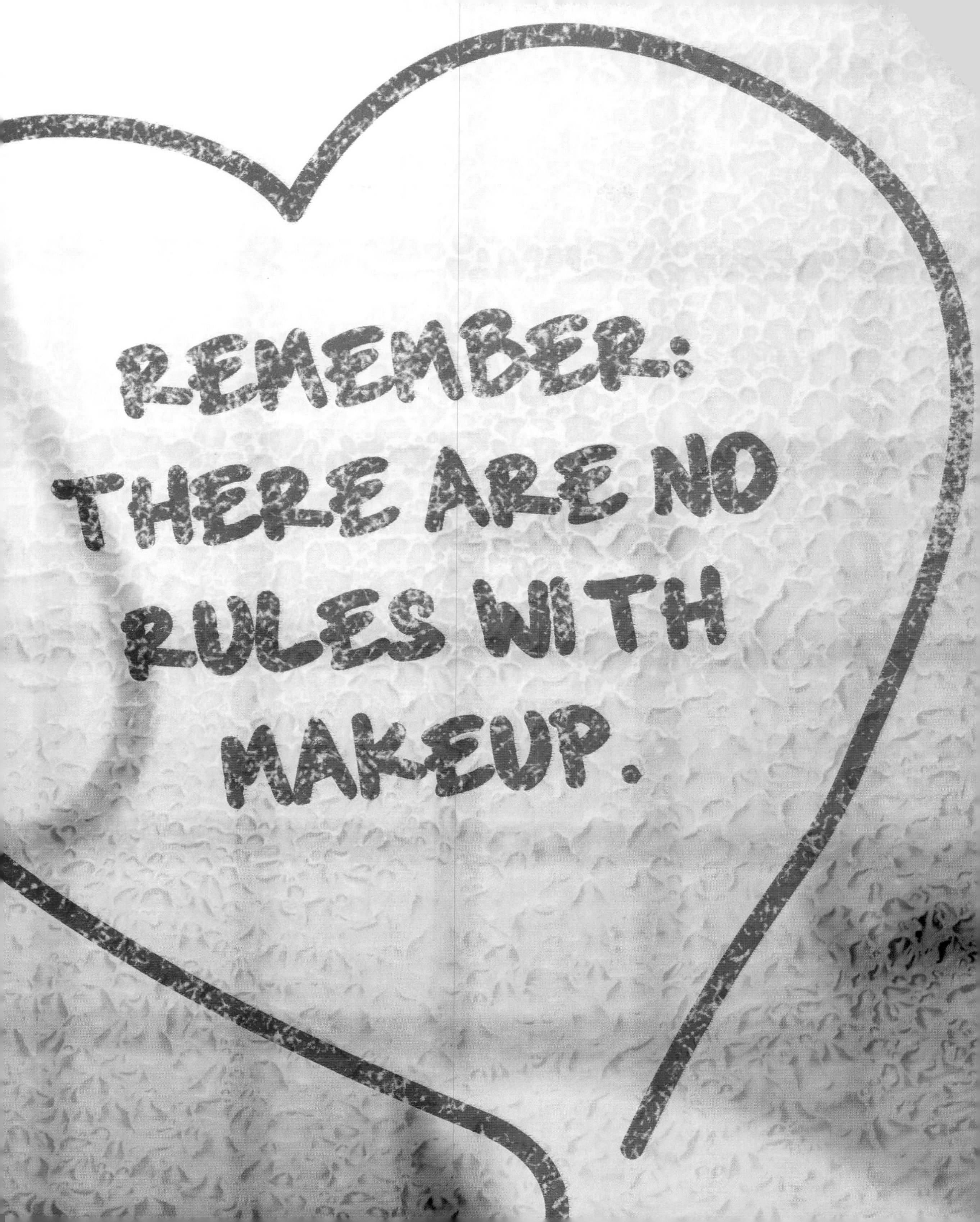
REMEMBER:
THERE ARE NO
RULES WITH
MAKEUP.

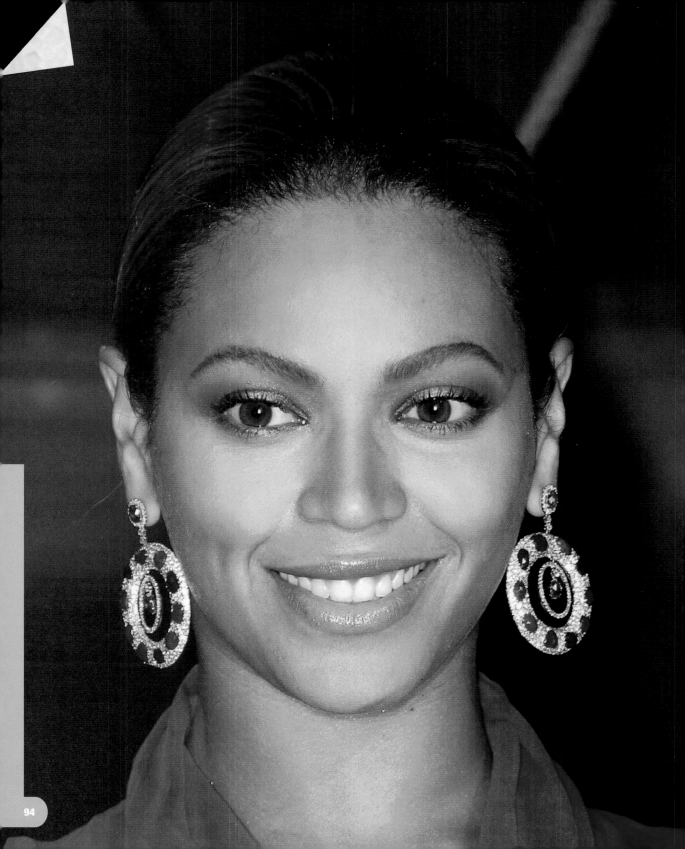

BEYONCÉ

VINTAGE GOLD

A **GORGEOUS**, GOLDEN BRONZE TOUCH THAT ADDS INTEREST TO THE **VINTAGE** LOOK.

THE PALETTE

* Ivory eye primer
* Dirty gold eyeshadow
* Metallic gold eyeshadow
* Dark brown frosted eyeshadow
* Golden bronze matte powder blush
* Frosted peach blush
* Pearlescent highlighter
* Powder foundation
* Black mascara
* Dark brown eyebrow powder

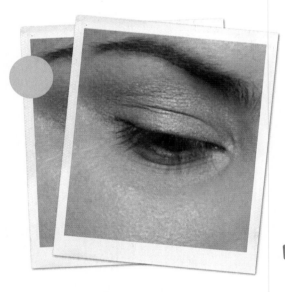

1. Use your third finger to apply ivory primer all over the eyelid and up to the brow.

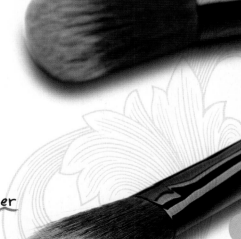

Using an eyeshadow brush, cover the entire eyelid and eyebrow area with **dirty gold** eyeshadow, creating a line from the outer corner of the eye up to the end of the eyebrow. Apply with a light touch.

Use a blender brush to gently feather the edge so there isn't a harsh line.

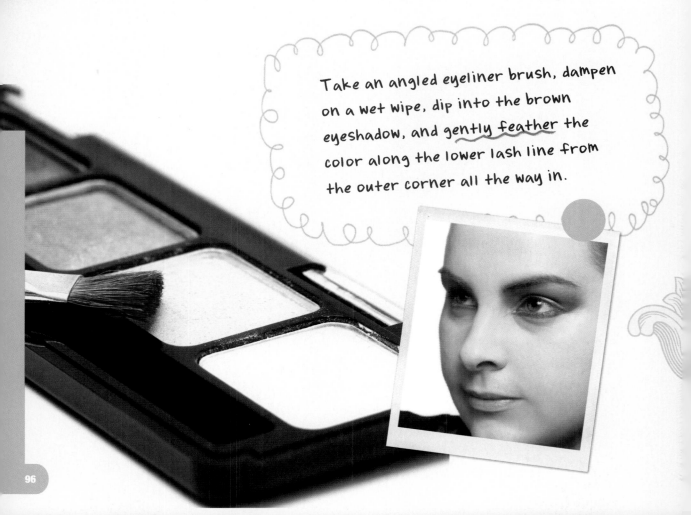

2. Now for the GOLD. Use an eyeshadow brush to gently pat metallic gold eyeshadow all over the eyelid to only a little way above the crease. Go right to the inner corner and out to just above the crease—don't extend the color.

Use a blender brush to apply dark brown frosted eyeshadow on the outer corner to just above the crease, over the gold, to add a little **depth**.

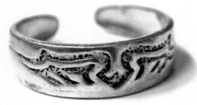

Take an angled eyeliner brush, dampen on a wet wipe, dip into the brown eyeshadow, and gently feather the color along the lower lash line from the outer corner all the way in.

Using the same brush, gently dab the metallic gold eyeshadow just above the brown all the way along the lower lash line.

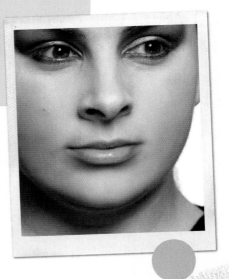

3. Use a **kabuki brush** to apply a golden bronze matte powder blush, sweeping it from the hairline, below the cheekbone, and under the chin.

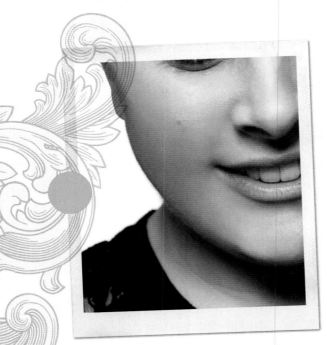

Then, with the same brush, gently flick a little frosted peach blush onto the cheekbone and up to the hairline.

With your finger gently dab pearlescent highlighter over the top of the cheekbone, adding a little along the nose.

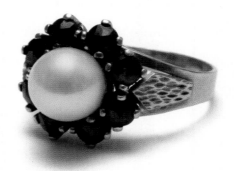

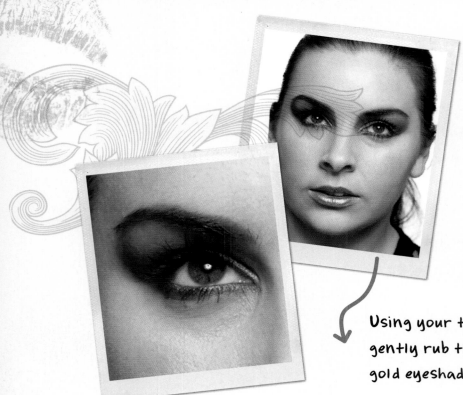

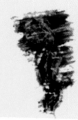

4. Use a foundation brush to apply a powder foundation all over the lips as a matte base.

Using your third finger, gently rub the same metallic gold eyeshadow over the lips.

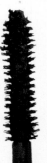

Tilt your head back and apply black mascara **lavishly** in an upwards and outwards motion. Add a touch to the bottom lashes.

Use a **Square** eyeliner brush to apply dark brown eyebrow powder to darken the eyebrows.

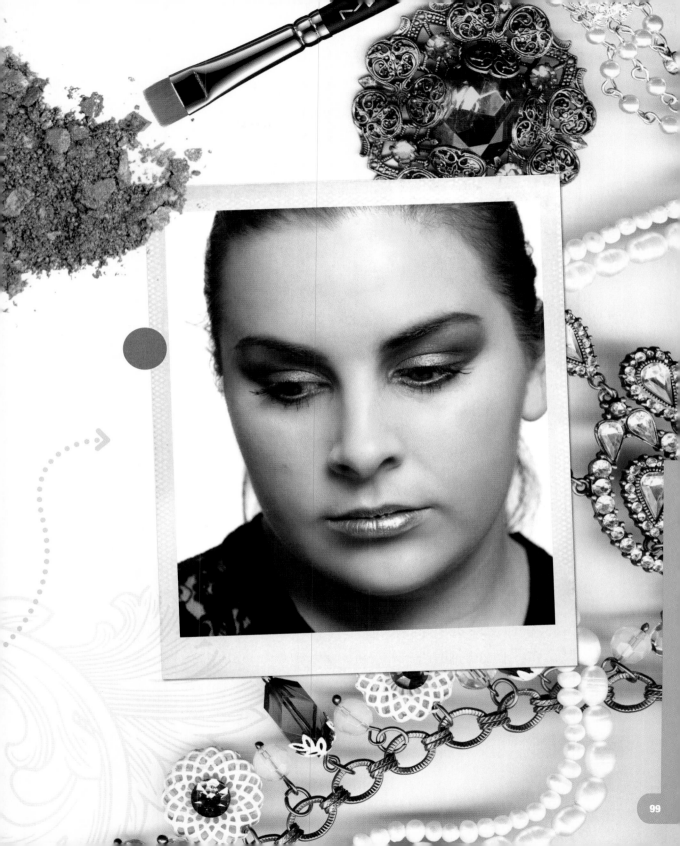

VINTAGE PRINCESS

OLD-FASHIONED GLAMOUR

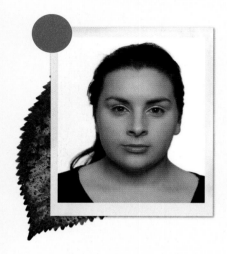

THIS IS A LOOK FOR **PALE SKIN**. IT'S REGAL WITH RICH TONES OF RED AND GOLD. WITH **STRONG** LIPSTICK, IT'S A GOOD AUTUMN LOOK, AND VERY MUCH FOR NOW. I LOVE IT.

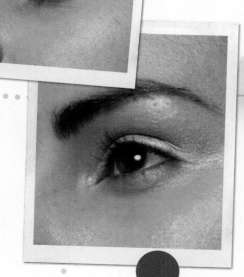

1. Cover the eyelid with a skin-colored cream primer, going right up to the eyebrow.

Use an eyeshadow brush to apply ivory eyeshadow all over the upper eyelid, starting from the middle. Pat it into the inner corner, up to the crease, and take it slightly beyond the outer edge onto the bone. Blend well.

THE PALETTE

* Skin-colored cream eye primer
* Ivory frosted eyeshadow
* Antique rust frosted eyeshadow
* Dark brown matte eyeshadow
* Black mascara
* Dark burgundy-brown lip liner
* Rich brick-red-brown lipstick
* Gold eyeshadow

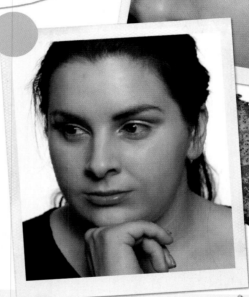

2. Tilt your head back. Use a blender brush to apply the antique rust eyeshadow along the crease line, back and forth, extending slightly onto the bone to cover the ivory eyeshadow.

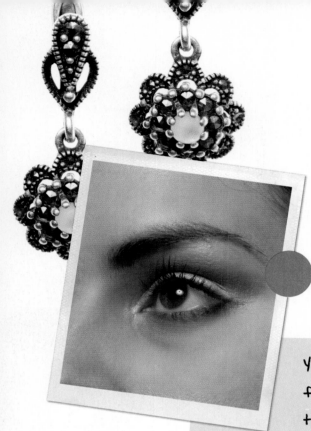

3. Dampen an angled eyeliner brush on a wet wipe. Take a little of the dark brown eyeshadow and, starting from the outer corner, work along the lower lash line two-thirds of the way in. Feather the color and make the line a little thicker at the outer corner.

You need very little black mascara for this look. Just a touch on the upper lashes.

4. Now for the lips. Using a dark burgundy-brown lip liner, draw slightly beyond the natural lip line, top and bottom, right to the corners.

Fill in with a rich brick-red-brown lipstick.

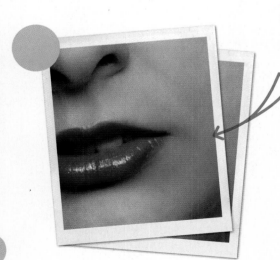

Finish by dabbing a little gold eyeshadow onto the center of the bottom lip. Gently rub the lips together to set the color.

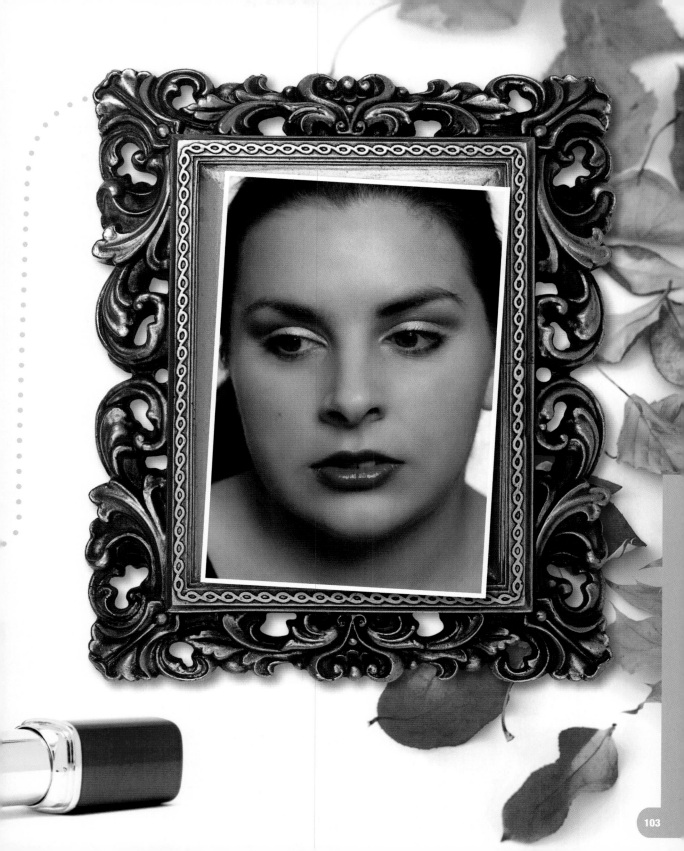

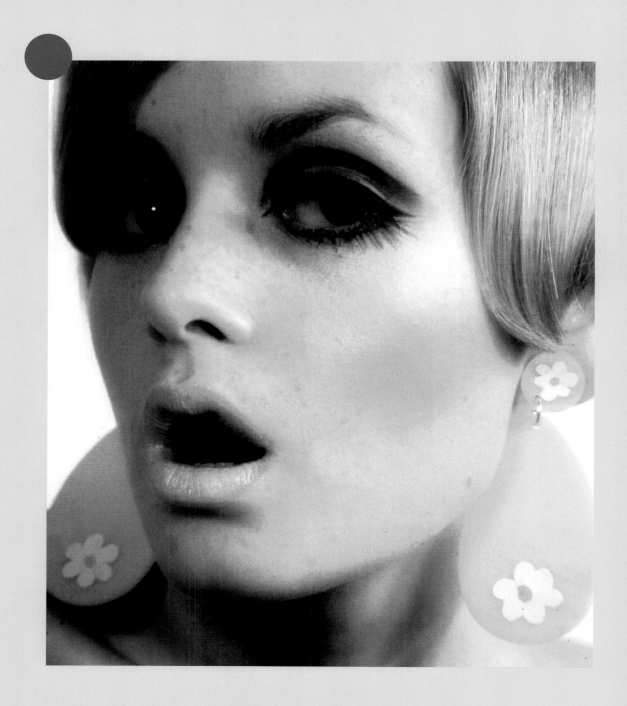

TWIGGY—MOD CON

1960S PIXIE

THE EYES ARE THE FOCAL POINT FOR THIS LOOK. THE ONLY THING YOU WANT TO STAND OUT ARE YOUR RAPUNZEL LASHES.

THINK DAISY CHAINS / HIPPIES— BACK WHEN THE WORLD WAS HAPPY.

THE PALETTE

* Golden brown matte bronzer
* Beige eye primer
* White frosted eyeshadow
* Black liquid eyeliner
* White eyeliner pencil
* Black mascara
* Foundation powder
* Pale lilac-pink matte lipstick

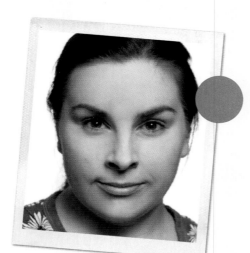

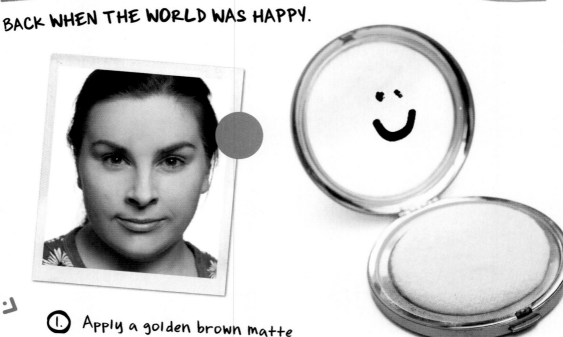

1. Apply a golden brown matte bronzer with a kabuki brush, moving from the ear onto the cheekbone and below. Use a circular motion, as if you are hollowing out your cheeks.

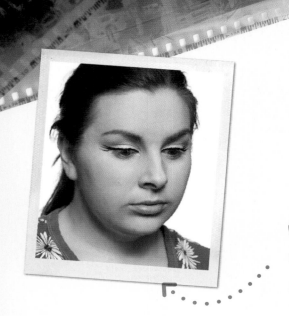

2. With your third finger, apply a beige eye primer all over the eyelid right up to the eyebrow bone.

Using an eyeshadow brush, dab white FROSTED EYESHADOW all over the eyelid, to just above the crease.

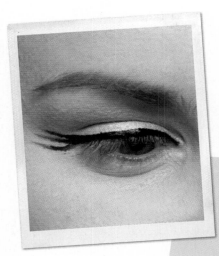

Apply black liquid eyeliner from the middle of the upper eyelid, working out and finishing with a **generous tick** at the outer corner. Then apply eyeliner from the inner corner, meeting in the middle.

If you are finding it tricky, use an angled eyeliner brush to apply rather than the applicator.

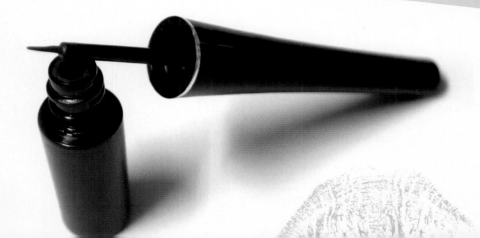

3. From near the outer edge, draw another line above and parallel to the tick so you now have two ticks.

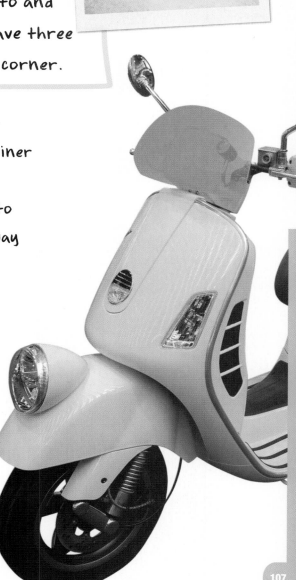

Then draw a third line parallel to and below the first tick. You now have three lines extending from the outer corner.

Now for the lower lashes, which are painted on with the black liquid eyeliner and the same angled eyeliner brush. Use your natural lashes as a guide to paint in eyelash lines most of the way along the lower eyelid.

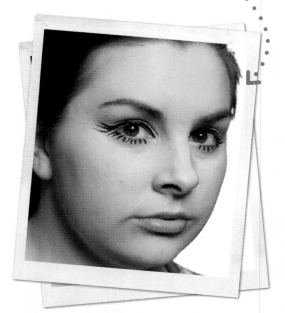

4. Run a white eyeliner pencil along the water line (see page 29) of the lower lashes.

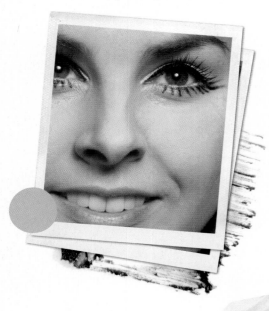

Apply black mascara to the upper lashes, wiggling the wand as you go upwards and then outwards.

5. Apply foundation powder to the lips as a matte base. Use a pale lilac-pink matte lipstick on both lips.

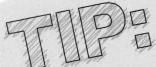

TIP:

If you want a thinner line for your "fake" lashes, hold the skin beneath the eye with two fingers slightly separated and let the eyeliner dry before you let go. This way, it won't bleed into the skin and thicken the lines.

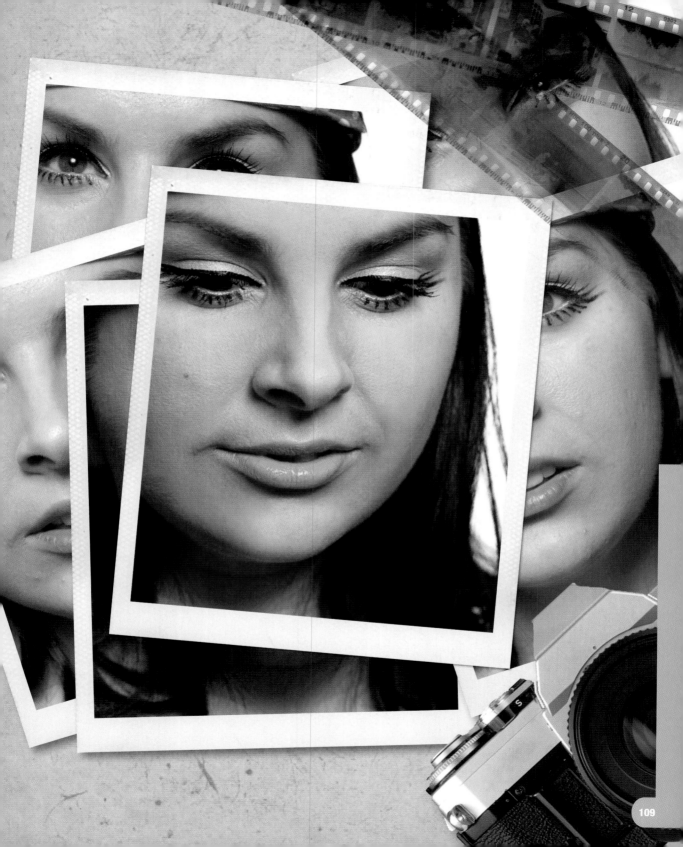

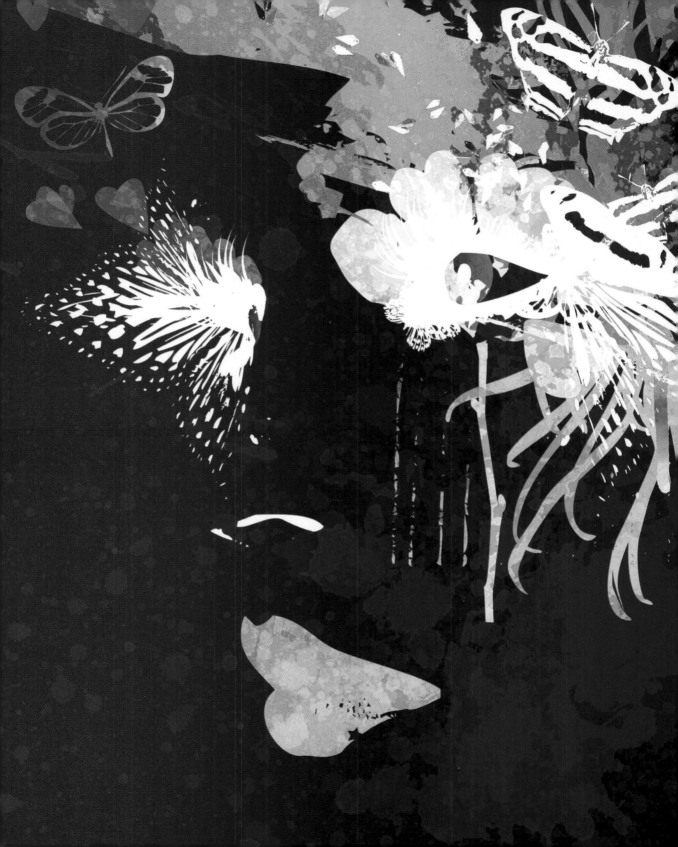

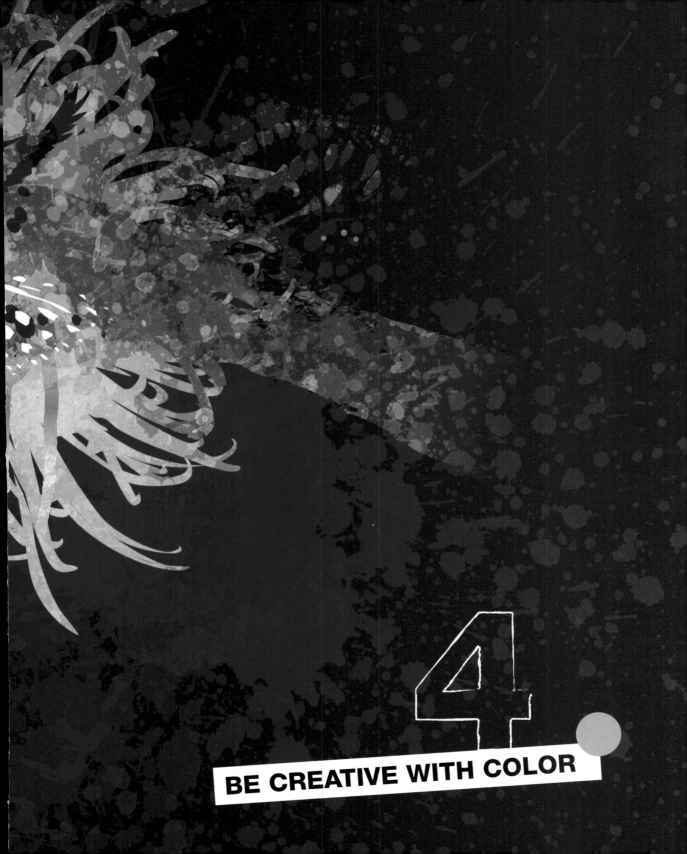

4

BE CREATIVE WITH COLOR

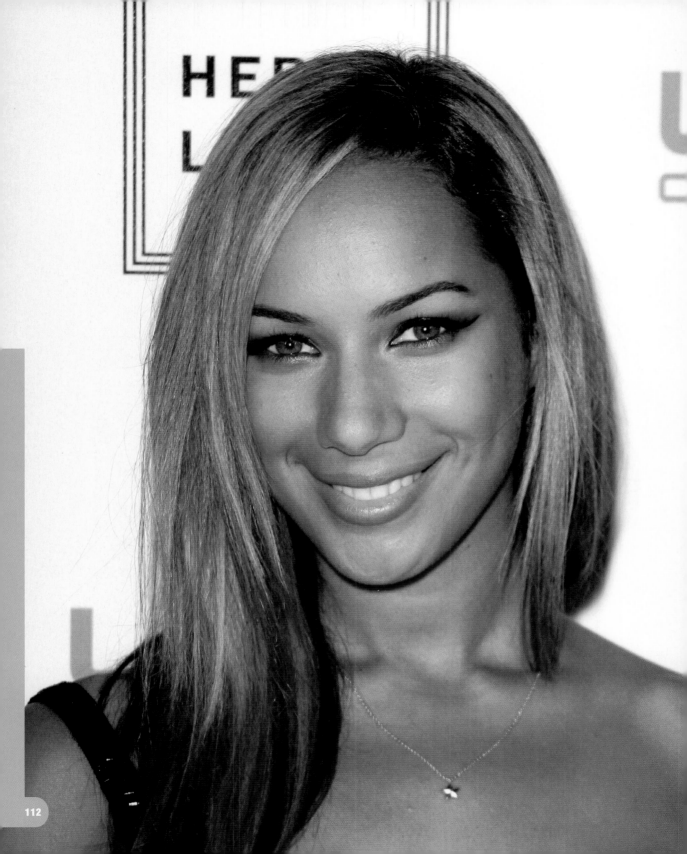

LEONA LEWIS
SMOLDERING SUPERSTAR

SMOKY DOESN'T HAVE TO BE JUST GRAY, BLACK, OR BROWN—IT CAN BE COLORFUL, TOO. HERE IT IS—GORGEOUS GREEN ALL THE WAY.

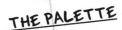

THE PALETTE

* Black creamy eyeshadow
* Dark smoky green frosted eyeshadow
* Light green frosted eyeshadow
* Black creamy eyeliner pencil
* White frosted eyeshadow
* Plum-pink satin lipstick
* Light coffee lip gloss

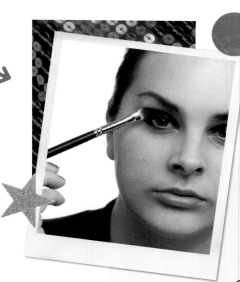

1. For this look you have to build up LAYERS OF COLOR, starting with black as the primer. Use an eyeshadow brush to apply BLACK CREAMY EYESHADOW all over the eyelid and outwards to create a tiny tick at the outer corner, going straight across from the crease (it should be squared off at the outer edge rather than tapered).

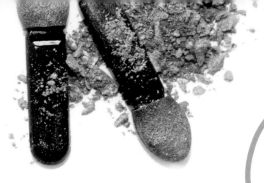

It looks a bit scary at this stage, but the black base holds the colors well and gives the exact shade of green I am after.

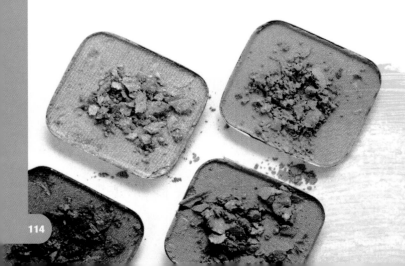

Now use an ANGLED EYELINER BRUSH and the same black eyeshadow to draw a line along the bottom from the middle to the outer corner, and then from the center to the inner corner. Make the line thicker at the outer corner and taper it gradually as you go in.

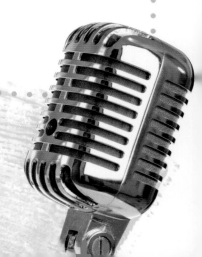

② Now for the greens. Using an EYESHADOW BRUSH, pat the DARK FROSTED GREEN EYESHADOW gently onto the black base and blend in well. Go right into the lash line so you don't end up with a gap.

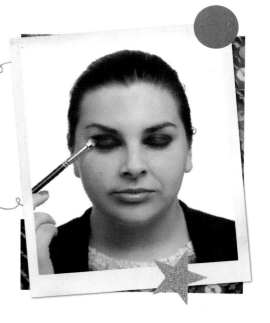

Using the eyeliner brush, cover the black base line along the lower lashes with the green, going right to the inner corner.

Use a CLEAN EYESHADOW BRUSH to apply the light green frosted eyeshadow over the dark green. Start from the outer corner of the eyelid and blend with the dark green, up and along the crease line, back and forth, to the inner eye.

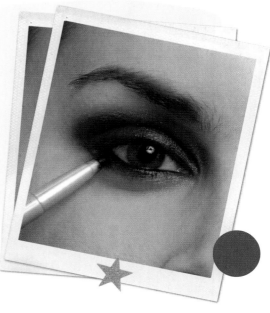

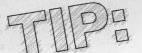

TIP:

USE A BLACK CREAMY EYELINER PENCIL ALONG THE LOWER LASH WATER LINE (THE WET PART) TO DEFINE THE EYES EVEN MORE.

③ Now for some **highlighter** to lift the colors. Use an eyeshadow brush to apply a frosted white eyeshadow under the eyebrows and down along the inside of the nose, filling in the entire area above the color.

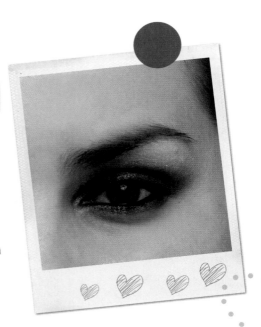

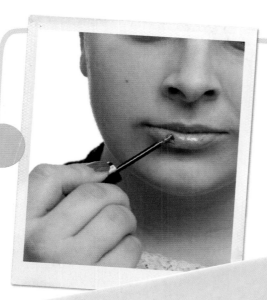

④ Apply a little mascara on the upper and lower lashes—you don't need too much.

⑤ Finish with a plum-pink lipstick and a light coffee lip gloss to give a nice juicy look to the lips.

TIP:

P.S. DON'T FORGET TO CHECK YOUR EYEBROWS. THEY MAY NEED TO BE TOUCHED UP WITH A DARK PENCIL OR EYEBROW POWDER SINCE THIS IS A VERY STRONG LOOK.

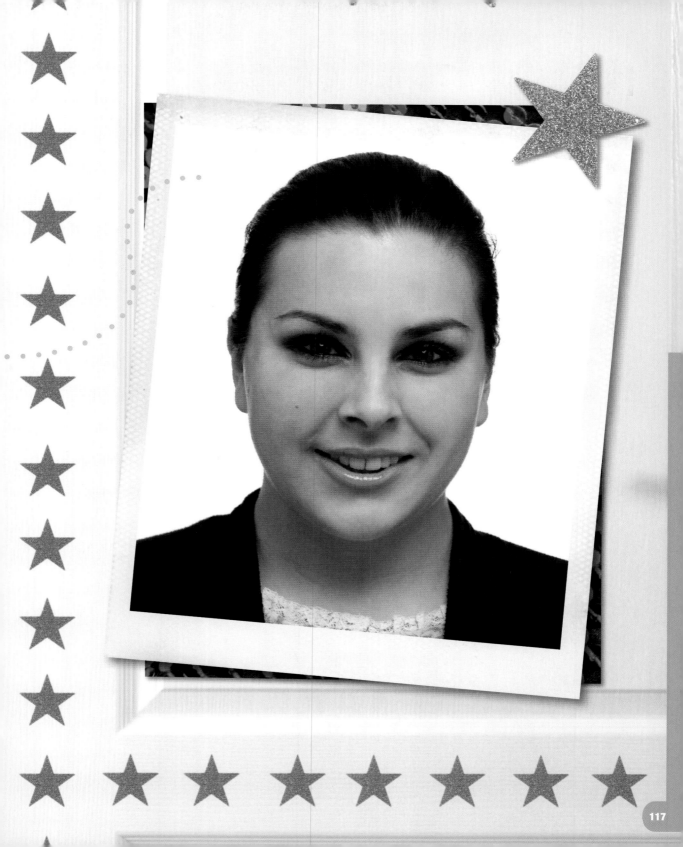

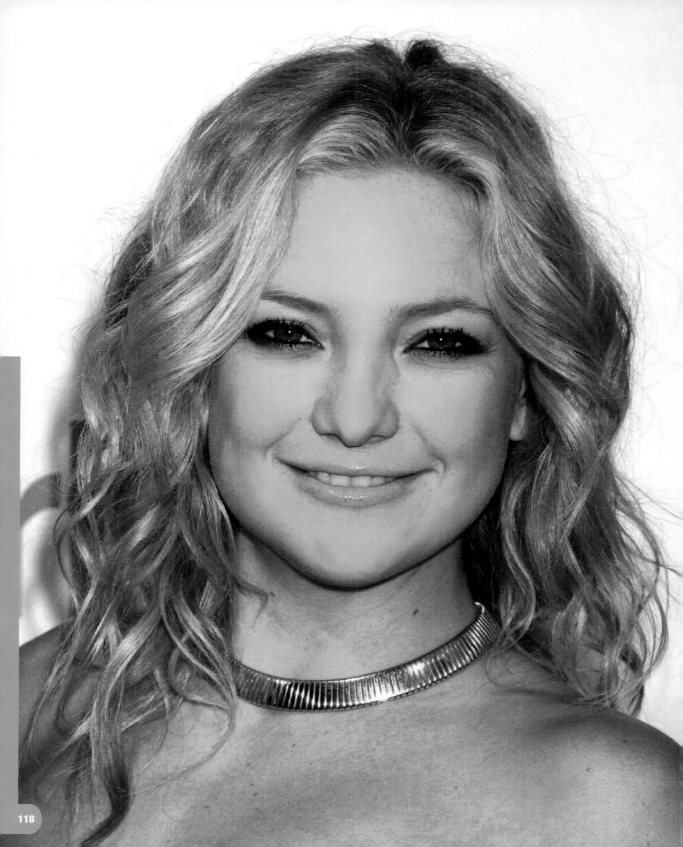

SUMMER GODDESS

GO FOR GOLD

DON'T BE SCARED OF
USING GOLD. IT LOOKS
INCREDIBLE HERE ON
KATE HUDSON, AND IS SO
COMPLEMENTARY—FOR
ALL EYE COLORS.

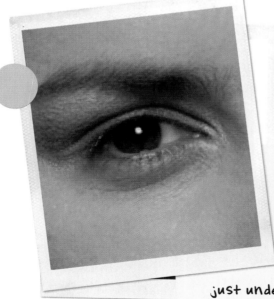

1. Prime the eyelid right up to just under the eyebrow with a FROSTED IVORY PRIMER.

Using an eyeshadow brush, apply the YELLOW-GOLD EYESHADOW all over the eyelid. Dab it on gently, going to the inner corner just under the eyebrow, along the crease and over the whole eyelid, right down to the lashes.

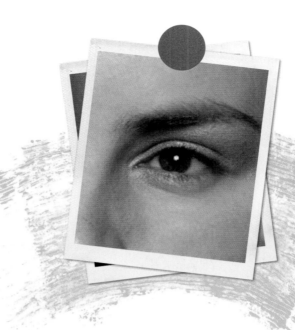

Use a fresh brush to gradually blend the color up to meet the eyebrow.

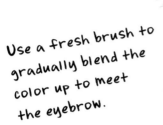

Using your ring finger, gently dab the white eyeshadow under the eyebrow and blend in well.

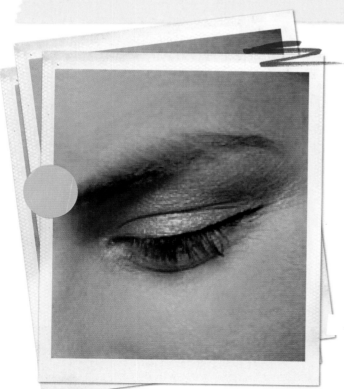

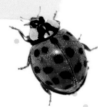

2. Rest the little finger on your cheek to keep your hand steady while you apply the eyeliner. Start in the middle of the upper eyelid and draw a very fine line to the outer corner, giving a little flick at the end.

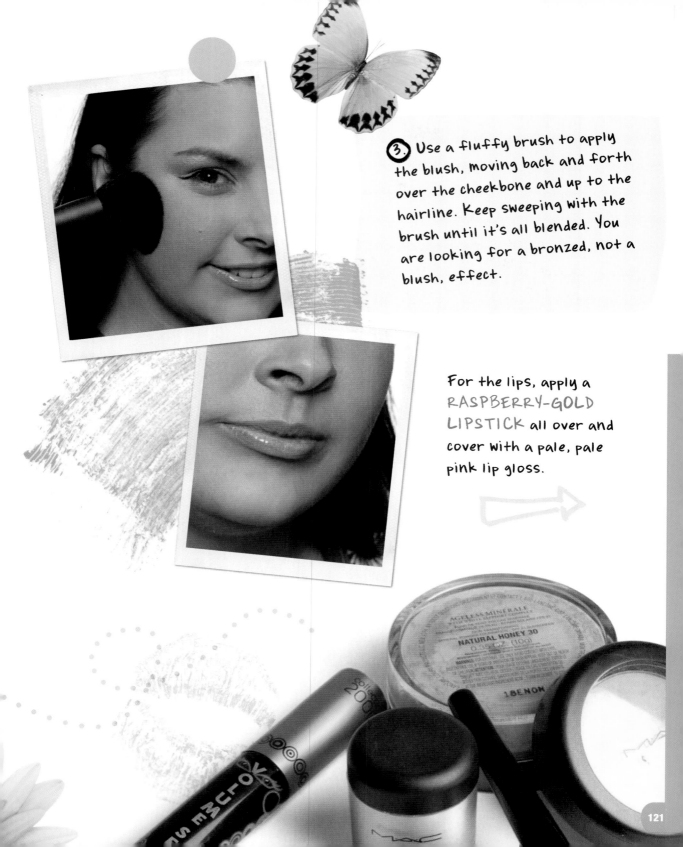

3. Use a fluffy brush to apply the blush, moving back and forth over the cheekbone and up to the hairline. Keep sweeping with the brush until it's all blended. You are looking for a bronzed, not a blush, effect.

For the lips, apply a RASPBERRY-GOLD LIPSTICK all over and cover with a pale, pale pink lip gloss.

④ Now take a honey-gold eyeliner pencil and, steadying your little finger on your cheek, start drawing a line from the outer corner of the lower lashes to the inner corner.

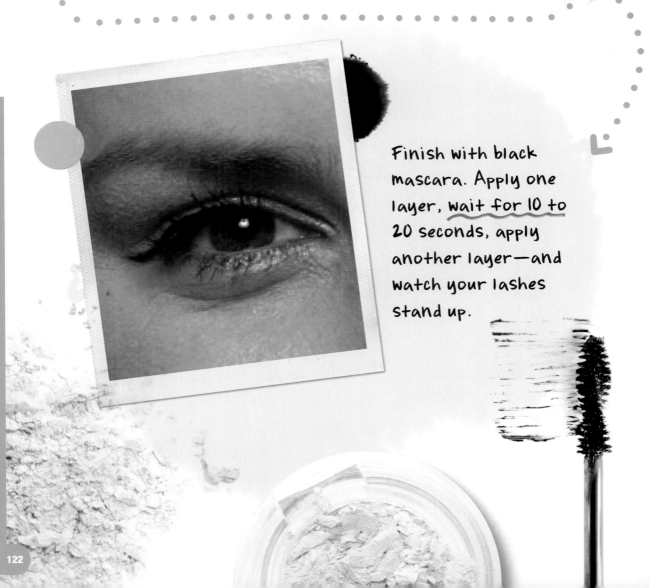

Finish with black mascara. Apply one layer, wait for 10 to 20 seconds, apply another layer—and watch your lashes stand up.

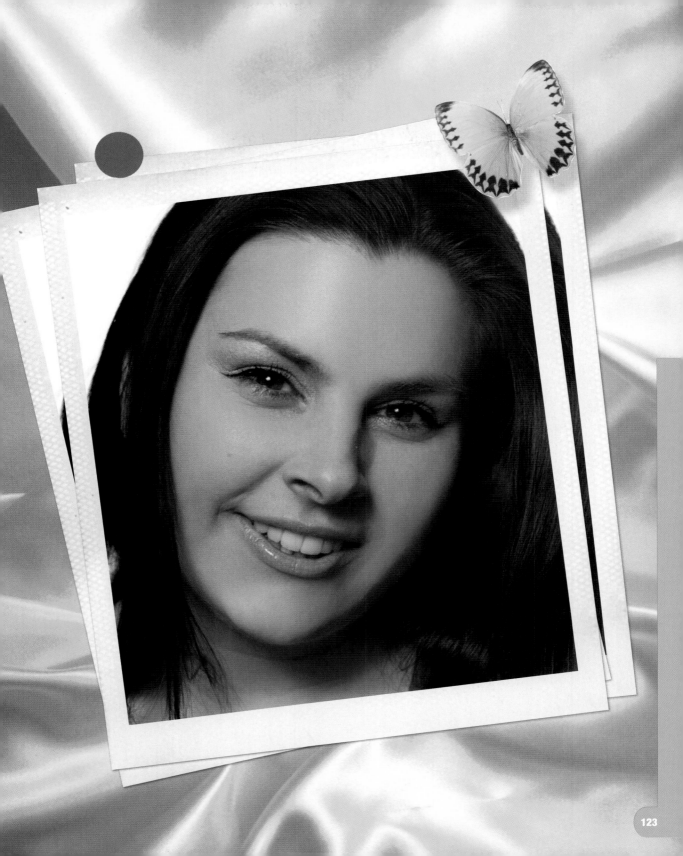

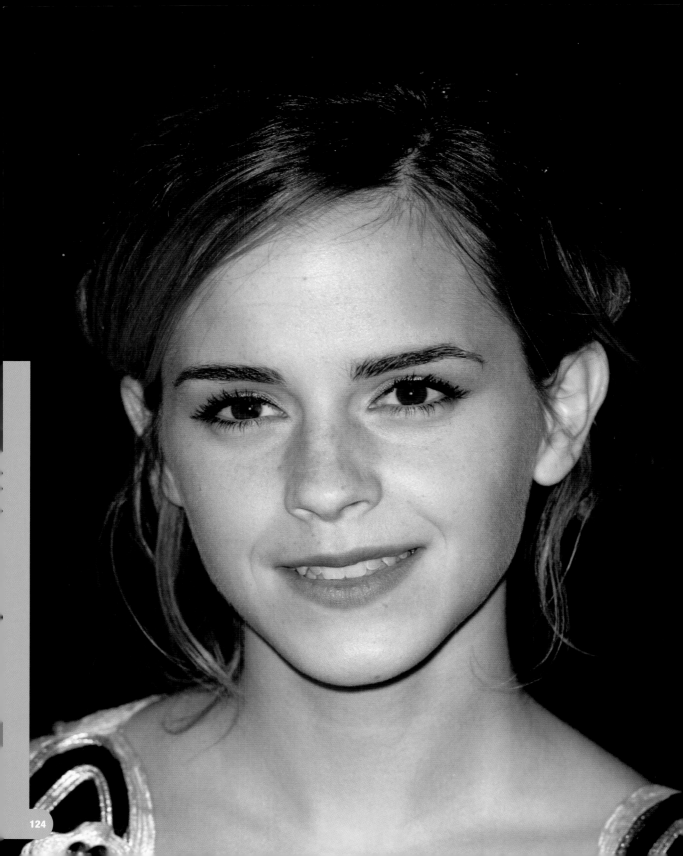

CUTE SPRINGTIME BEAUTY

SOFT AND DEWY

LIKE EMMA WATSON, THIS LOOK WILL MAKE YOU LOOK FRESH AS A DAISY —SIMPLE, SHIMMERING GORGEOUSNESS.

THE PALETTE

* Black creamy eyeshadow
* Dark smoky green frosted eyeshadow
* Light green frosted eyeshadow
* Black creamy eyeliner pencil
* White frosted eyeshadow
* Plum-pink satin lipstick
* Light coffee lip gloss

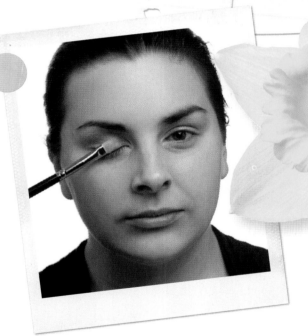

1 Use your third finger to apply a beige eye primer, from the lashline up to the eyebrow.

Using an eyeshadow brush, apply white eyeshadow from the middle of the eyelid down along the inside of the nose. This really opens up the eye.

Then, using the same brush, dampen it on a wet wipe and apply a little gold from the outer lash line to meet the white and blend the colors together.

Use an angled eyeliner brush to repeat the white and gold applications all the way along the lower lash line. Mix well to create lemon.

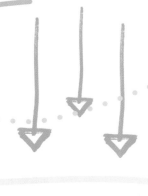

② Now for the orange. Use an eyeshadow brush to pat orange eyeshadow powder gently all over the outer corner of the eyelid, up past the crease, pushing into the inner corner of the eyebrow. Not too much—go gradually. The powder can easily fall off the brush onto your cheeks.

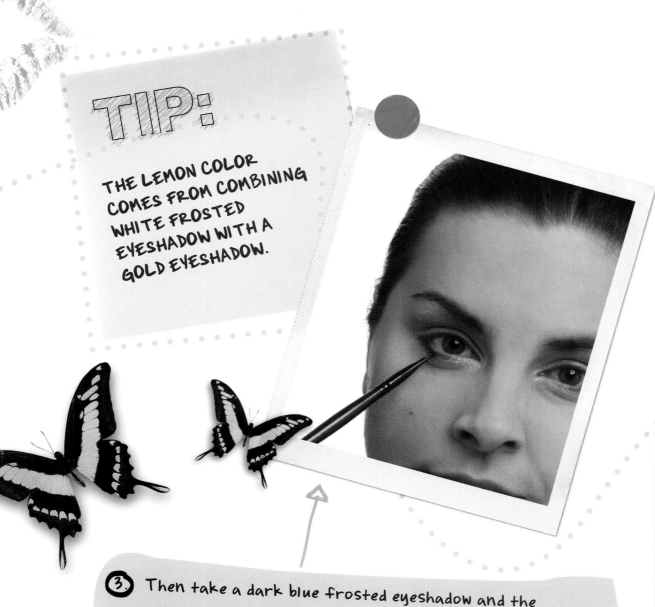

TIP:

THE LEMON COLOR COMES FROM COMBINING WHITE FROSTED EYESHADOW WITH A GOLD EYESHADOW.

3. Then take a dark blue frosted eyeshadow and the angled eyeliner brush. Rest your little finger on your cheek to steady your hand. Start from the outer corner, bring the color a quarter of the way in, fading gradually, and blend with the gold roughly in the center of the eye. Take it out a little at the corner—this will complement and accentuate the shape of the eye.

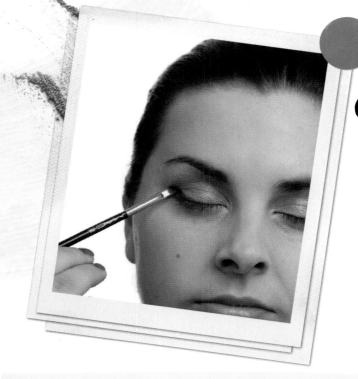

4. Use a wet wipe to clean the same angled eyeliner brush. Make sure the brush line is nice and sharp. Gently hold the eyelid shut, and apply chocolate-brown eyeshadow from halfway across the upper lash line, in a fine line to the outer corner and just beyond. Blend up and into the orange.

Keep blending—you don't want too much. If you have overdone it, smooth off any excess with your finger or go back over it again with the orange and carry on blending. Mistakes do happen—all the time!

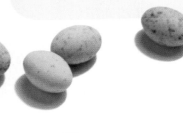

5 Apply a little mascara on the upper and lower lashes.

I like a pink cream blusher for this look. Use your third finger to dot it onto the cheeks and blend well.

Then gently dot a pearlescent highlighter on your cheeks, coming up and around the outer edge of the eye in a C motion. If you like, you can put a little on your nose and chin, though I find that makes me look too shiny.

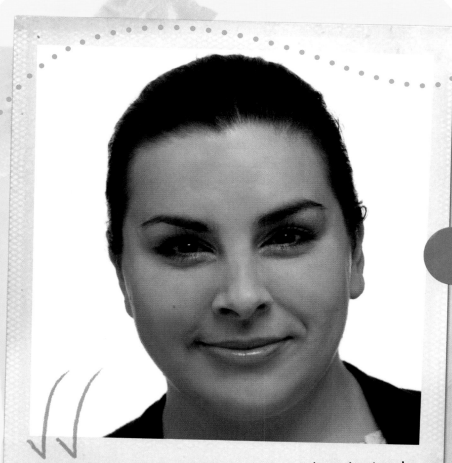

Finish with a dark coffee satin lipstick and a touch of light coffee lip gloss on the lower lip only.

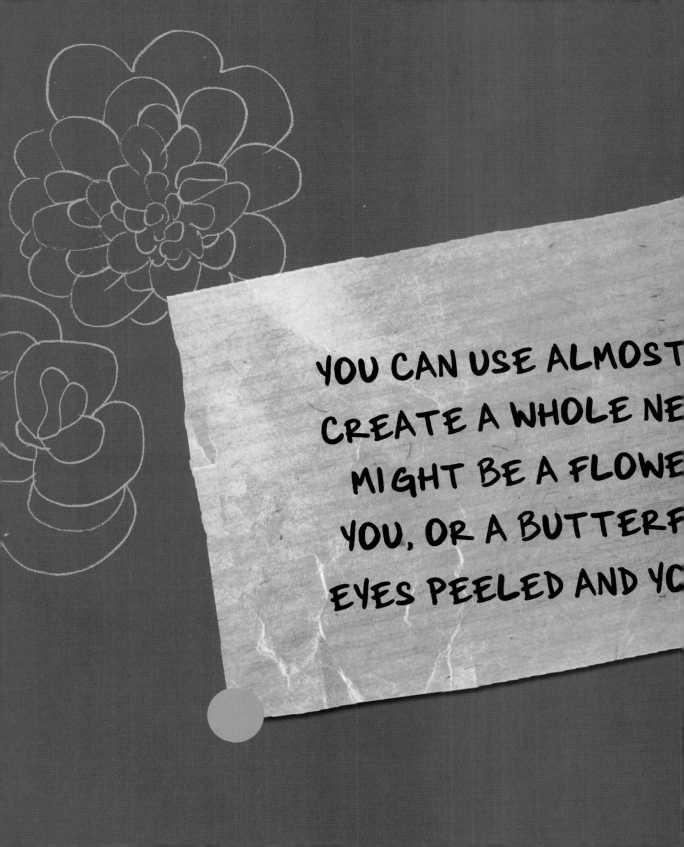

YOU CAN USE ALMOST
CREATE A WHOLE NE
MIGHT BE A FLOWE
YOU, OR A BUTTERF
EYES PEELED AND YO

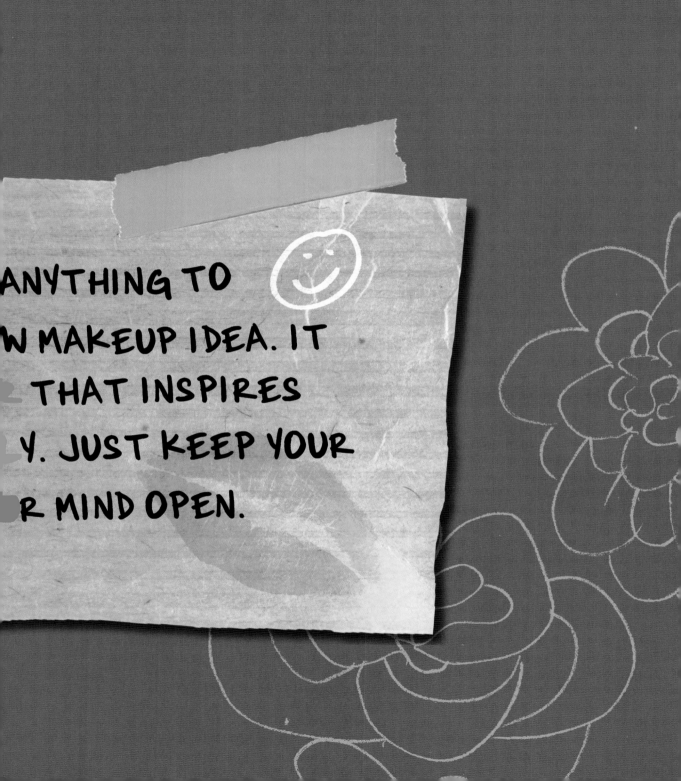

ANYTHING TO

W MAKEUP IDEA. IT

THAT INSPIRES

Y. JUST KEEP YOUR

R MIND OPEN.

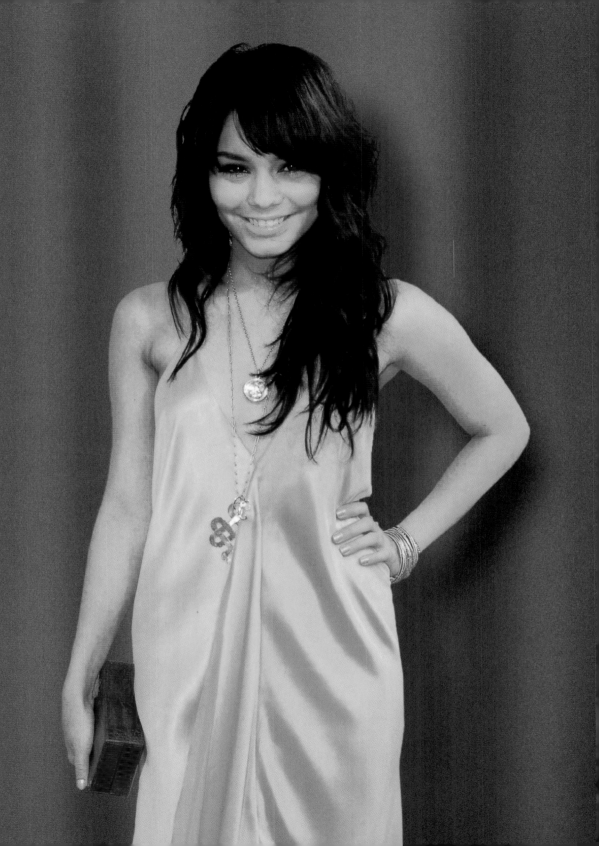

PROM

DANCING QUEEN

STAND OUT IN THE CROWD LIKE VANESSA HUDGENS WITH THIS BEAUTIFUL PURPLE PEARLESCENT LOOK. IT'S YOUR SPECIAL NIGHT —ENJOY IT!

THE PALETTE

* Purple cream eyeshadow or shadestick
* Frosted lavender eyeshadow
* Pearlescent white eyeshadow
* Light pink frosted blush
* Matte plum-pink lip liner pencil
* Matte cherry-pink lipstick
* Black mascara

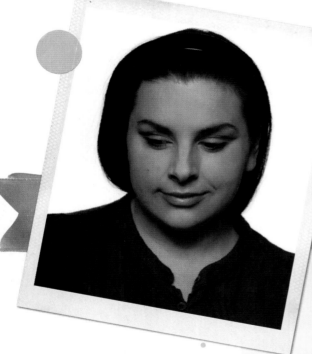

1. Prime the eye with a purple eyeshadow or shadestick.

Take the purple from the inner corner, along and slightly above the crease, going to the outer corner and finishing with a slight tick (you are not covering the eyelid).

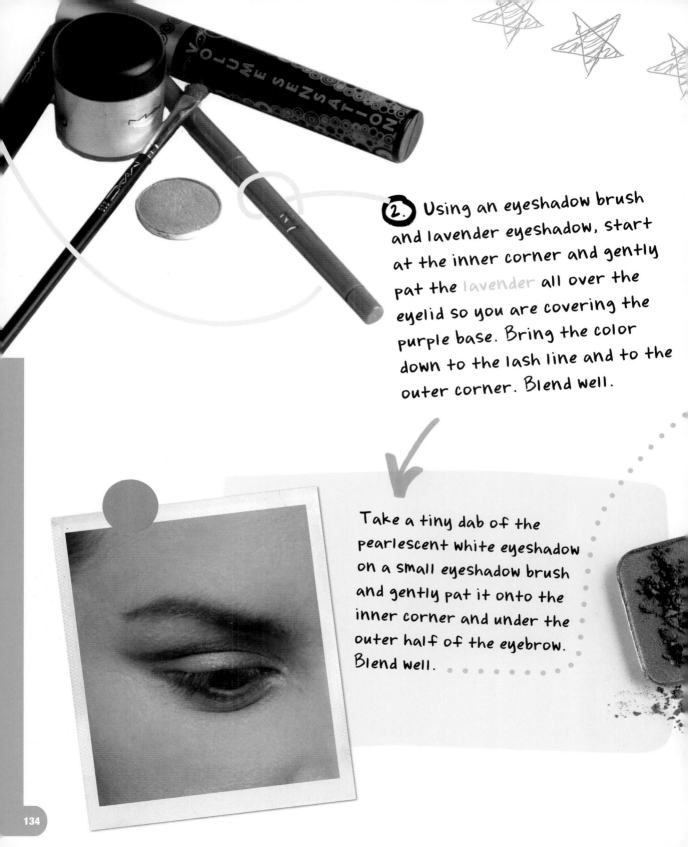

2. Using an eyeshadow brush and lavender eyeshadow, start at the inner corner and gently pat the lavender all over the eyelid so you are covering the purple base. Bring the color down to the lash line and to the outer corner. Blend well.

Take a tiny dab of the pearlescent white eyeshadow on a small eyeshadow brush and gently pat it onto the inner corner and under the outer half of the eyebrow. Blend well.

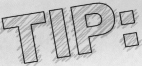

I AM USING PURPLE AS THE BASE FOR THIS LOOK BECAUSE THE COLOR WILL SHOW THROUGH THE PALER LAVENDER EYESHADOW THAT IS APPLIED ON TOP.

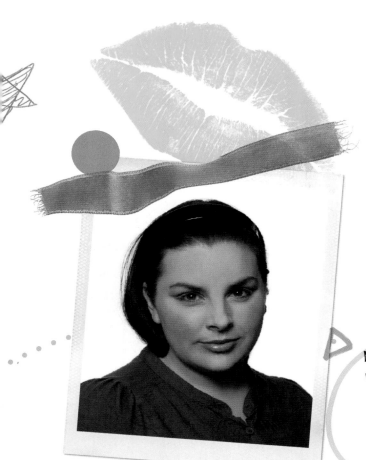

Now, with an angled eyeliner brush, add a touch of the purple base to the lower lash line. Start at the outer corner and work in about two-thirds of the way, and feather to blend in and soften the effect.

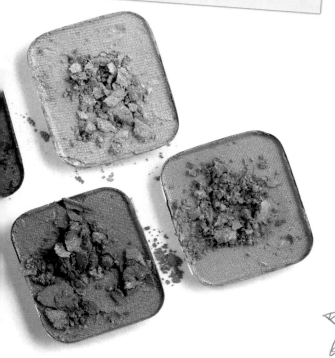

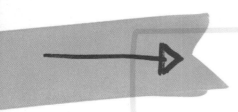

3 **Smile,** and use a fluffy brush to apply a generous amount of light pink blush to the apple of the cheek. Blend the color well in a circular motion.

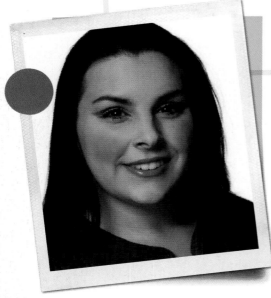

With a matte plum-pink lip liner pencil, draw a line from the Cupid's bow to the outer corners. Rest the little finger on the chin and rock the pencil back and forth on the lower lip, moving from the center to the outer corners.

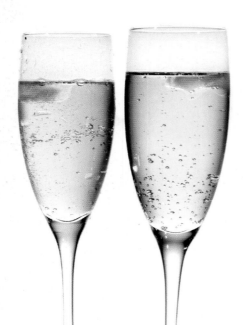

Fill the lips in with a matte cherry-pink lipstick.

Finish with a touch of black mascara on the upper and lower lashes.

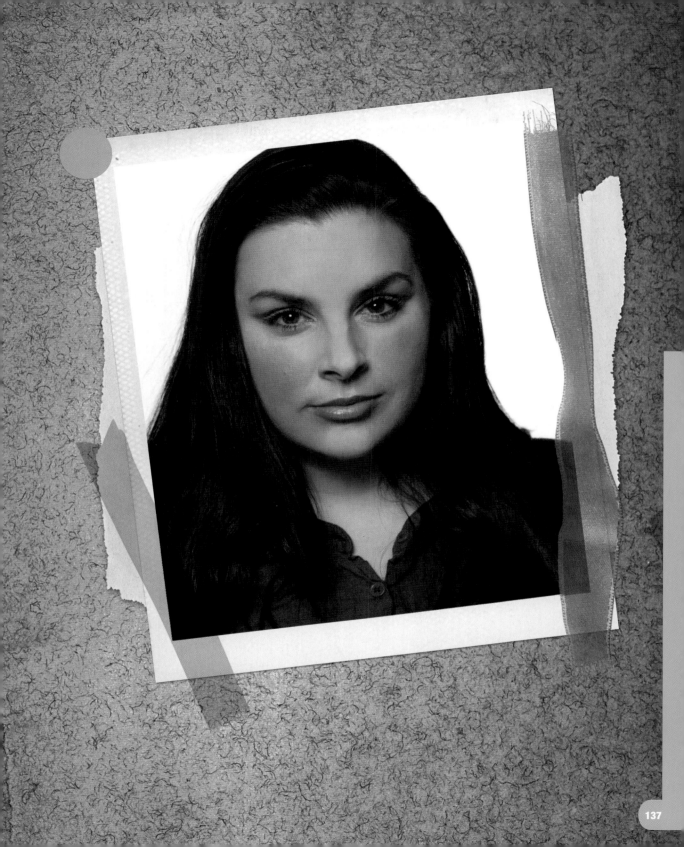

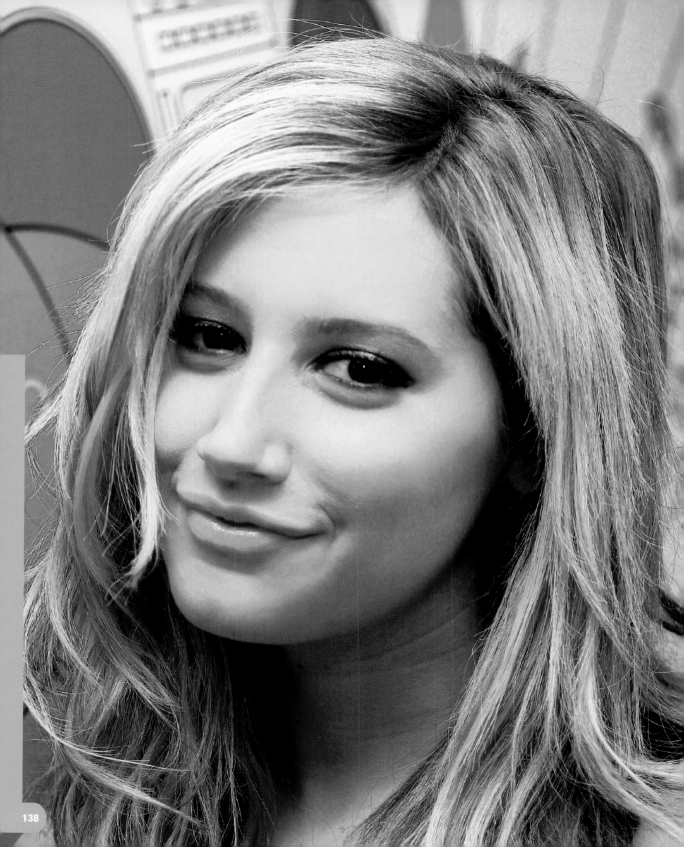

ASHLEY TISDALE

GIRLS NIGHT OUT

THIS IS A SMOKY BLUE LOOK, USING A RICH, DARK NAVY BLUE. IT'S GREAT FOR A NIGHT ON THE TOWN.

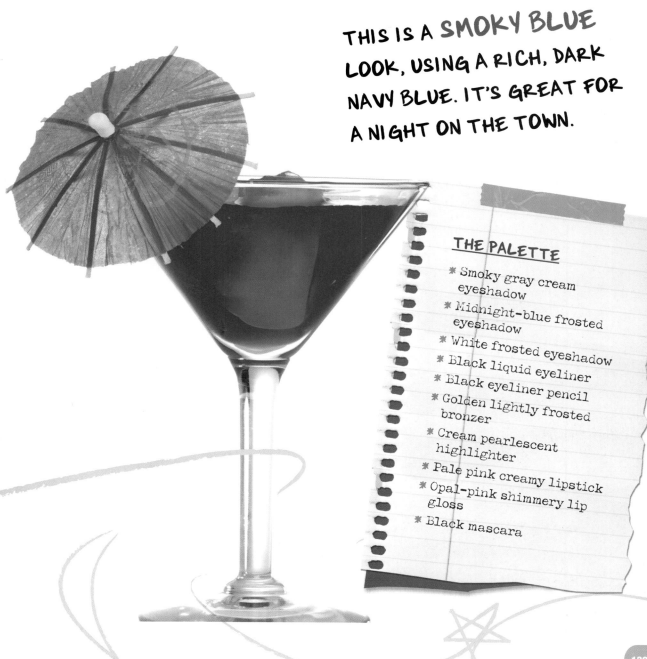

THE PALETTE

* Smoky gray cream eyeshadow
* Midnight-blue frosted eyeshadow
* White frosted eyeshadow
* Black liquid eyeliner
* Black eyeliner pencil
* Golden lightly frosted bronzer
* Cream pearlescent highlighter
* Pale pink creamy lipstick
* Opal-pink shimmery lip gloss
* Black mascara

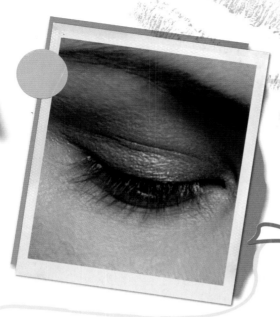

1. Using your third finger, apply smoky gray eyeshadow all over the eyelid and up just past the crease, going slightly beyond the outer edge. Blend in well.

2. Use a dampened angled eyeliner brush with the midnight blue eyeshadow and gently draw a line along the upper lashes from the inner to the outer corner, extending slightly at the outer edge. It will be a fairly thick line, so feather it with a sponge-tipped brush.

Now draw a line with the blue eyeshadow from halfway along the lower lashes, extending at the outer corner (we are keeping the inner corner for highlighting).

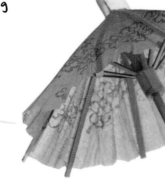

3 Use the sponge-tipped brush to dab a little white frosted eyeshadow on the inner corner of the upper and lower lids. Blend along to meet the blue.

Now carefully apply black liquid eyeliner on the outer half of the upper eyelid, over the blue line.

Then use a black creamy eyeliner pencil on the water line (see page 29) of the lower lash line.

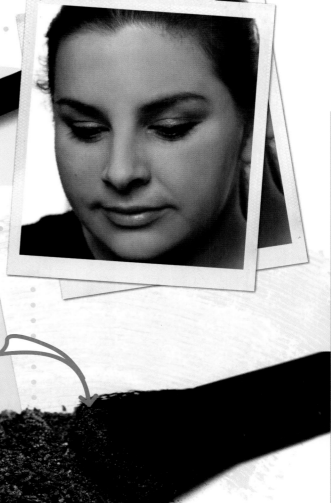

TIP:

BLUE EYESHADOW IS A STRONG COLOR AND IT TENDS TO FIND ITS WAY ONTO YOUR CHEEKS. KEEP CHECKING AND REMOVE ANY FALLOUT AS YOU GO.

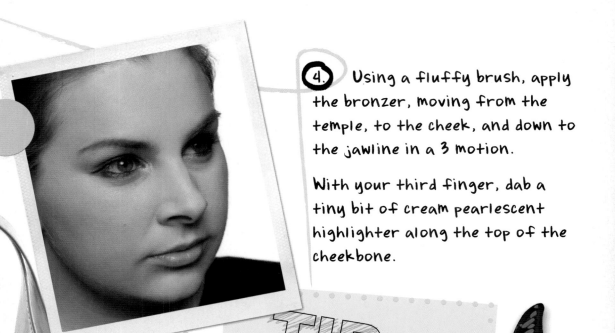

4. Using a fluffy brush, apply the bronzer, moving from the temple, to the cheek, and down to the jawline in a 3 motion.

With your third finger, dab a tiny bit of cream pearlescent highlighter along the top of the cheekbone.

TIP:

APPLYING EYELINER PENCIL ON THE WATER LINE DARKENS THE EYES AND GIVES A REALLY DRAMATIC EFFECT.

5. Prime the lips with a little foundation and then apply a very pale PINK CREAMY LIPSTICK.

Top with an opal-pink shimmery lip gloss and, if you want more of a glow, dab a little of the white highlighter in the middle of the top and bottom lips.

Apply black mascara to the upper and lower lashes, and you're ready to go.

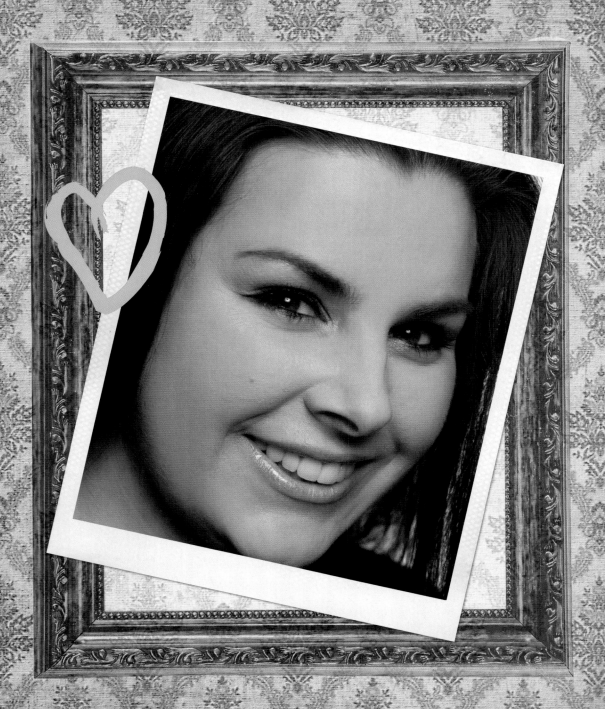

ROSEBUD BEAUTY

SOFT EYES AND A KISSABLE POUT

THIS IS A **SOFT** AND **INNOCENT** LOOK WITH COLORFUL, POUTY LIPS—IDEAL FOR GOING ON A PICNIC OR A FIRST DATE. IT USES A REALLY WACKY COLOR, BUT BECAUSE IT'S ONLY APPLIED TO THE INNER CORNER OF THE EYE, THE EDGE IS TAKEN OFF AND THE OVERALL EFFECT IS JUST BEAUTIFUL.

THE PALETTE

* Cream frosted eye primer
* Acid-green frosted eyeshadow
* Forest-green matte eyeshadow
* Plum-rosy-pink blush
* Black mascara
* Cranberry creamy lip liner
* Rosebud-pink lipstick with satin finish
* Nude lip gloss
* Black mascara
* Foundation
* Pale silvery-pink lipstick
* Light pink pearly lip gloss
* White frosted eyeshadow

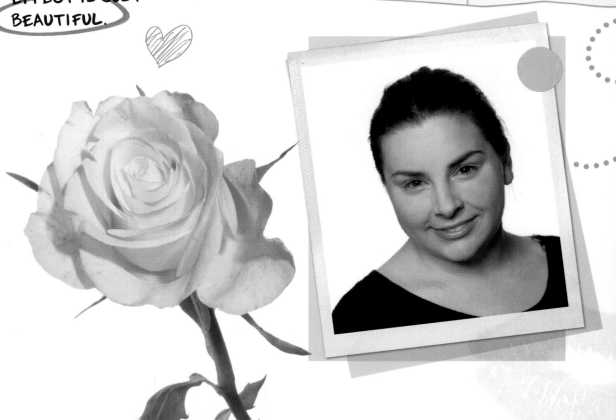

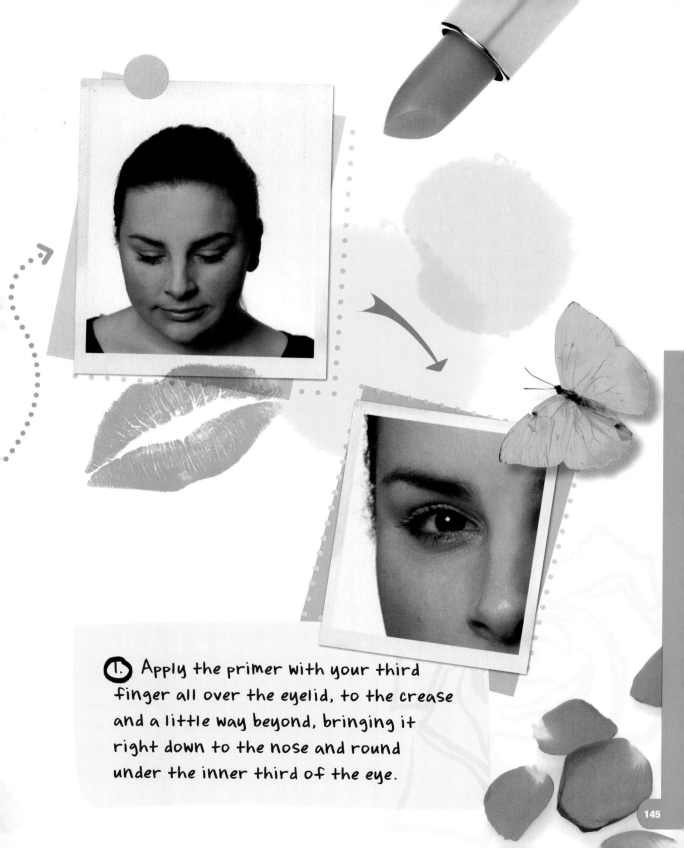

1. Apply the primer with your third finger all over the eyelid, to the crease and a little way beyond, bringing it right down to the nose and round under the inner third of the eye.

2 Dip an eyeshadow brush generously into the acid-green eyeshadow. You want a really powdered effect, and you will be focusing on the inner corner of the eye.

Starting at the inner corner, right by the nose, gently stroke the color two-thirds of the way along the upper eyelid, and then gently stroke it onto the lower lash line to cover the primer.

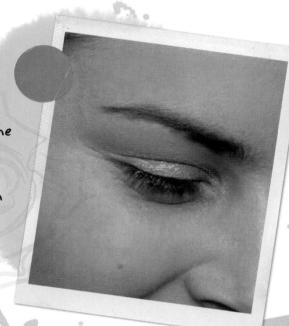

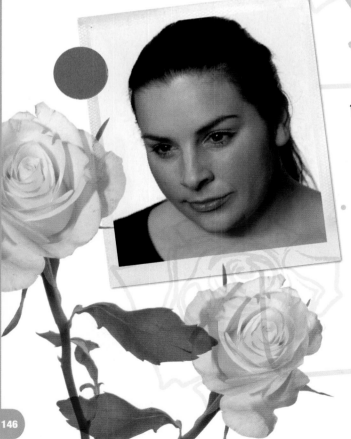

Blend the color out a little towards the outer corner of the upper eyelid, fading the color as you go.

Take an angled eyeliner brush and the forest-green eyeshadow. Start from the outer corner and gently join up to the acid green. Extend the line slightly at the outer corner. Blend well.

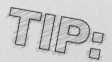

3 To get this slightly windswept look, you really need a plum to rosy-pink blush (no reds or peaches, please). Smile, and brush it onto the apple of the cheek, moving gently up to the hairline.

Add a layer of BLACK MASCARA on the upper lashes and a light touch on the lower lashes.

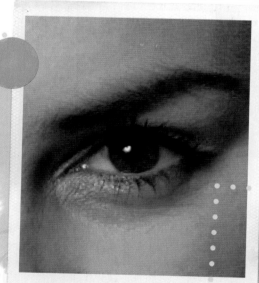

TIP:

APPLYING EYE PRIMER AROUND AND JUST BELOW THE INNER EYE AREA WILL REALLY CHANGE THE SHAPE OF YOUR EYES AND MAKE THEM LOOK FRESH AND OPEN.

4. Now for the grand finale—the lips. Using the cranberry lip liner, start with the Cupid's bow and gently fill it in to give the pouty look. Feather the color to the outer corners, very slightly above the natural lip line.

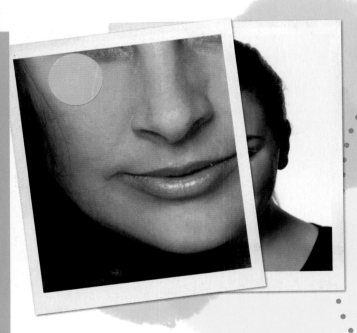

Make a line on the lower lip, very slightly below the natural lip line, but don't go into the corners. This makes the bottom lip look thicker as well.

Fill the lips in with a rosebud-pink satiny lipstick, and finish with a dab of natural lip gloss in the middle of the top and bottom lips.

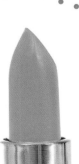
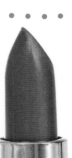
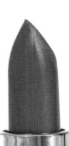
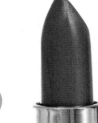

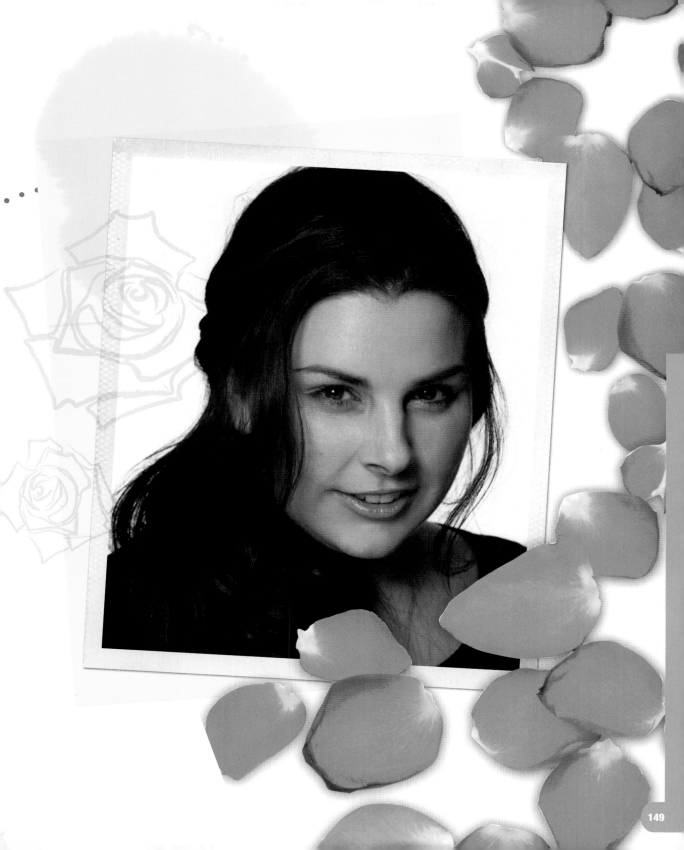

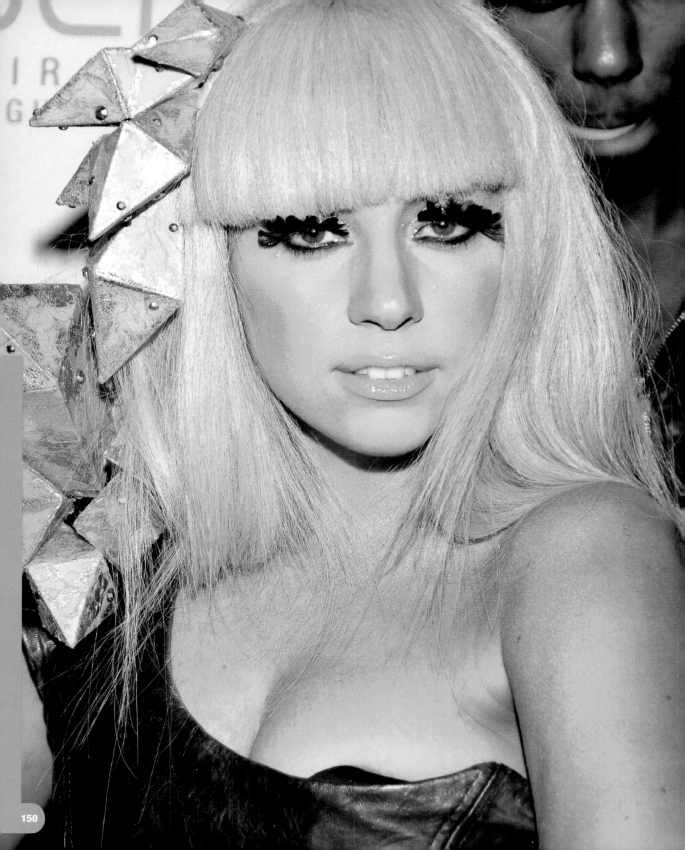

LADY GAGA

FIERCE AND FEARLESS

LADY GAGA REALLY KNOWS HOW TO PUSH A LOOK. SHE'S NOT AFRAID TO BE BOLD AND MAKE A STATEMENT WITH HER MAKEUP, AND NOR SHOULD YOU BE!

THE PALETTE

* Beige creamy eye primer
* Metallic silver pigment powder
* Baby-pink satin blush
* Ivory pearlescent highlighter
* Black creamy eyeliner pencil
* Black mascara
* Foundation
* Pale silvery-pink lipstick
* Light pink pearly lip gloss
* White frosted eyeshadow

1. Use your third finger to apply a beige creamy primer all over the eyelid and up to the eyebrow. Then run it along the lower lash line as well as right to the inner corner.

Use an eyeshadow brush to apply a metallic silver pigment powder. Start at the inner corner and dab it across the eyelid up to and just above the crease.

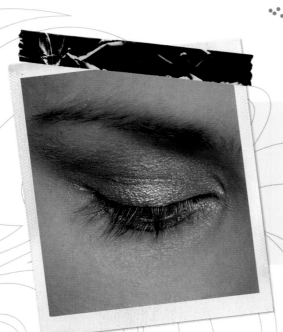

Dab it on the lower inner corner as well, and then take it all the way across the lower lash line.

2. With a fluffy brush, apply a light, baby-pink satin blush under the cheekbone to the jawline, moving in an up-and-down motion to the hairline.

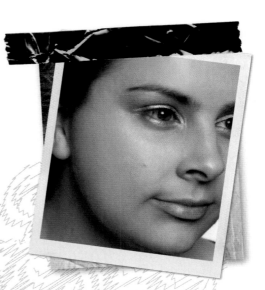

Using the same brush and an ivory pearlescent highlighter, start across the forehead, moving down along and underneath the nose to the chin. Then onto the cheekbone, just above the blush and up to the hairline.

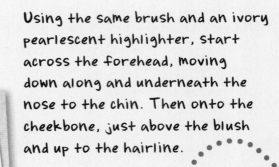

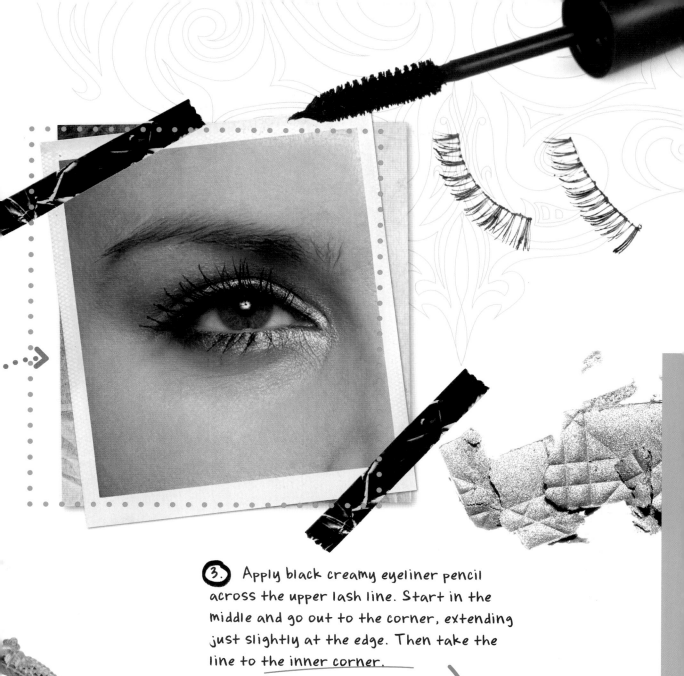

3. Apply black creamy eyeliner pencil across the upper lash line. Start in the middle and go out to the corner, extending just slightly at the edge. Then take the line to the <u>inner corner</u>.

Draw a line along the lower lashes from the outer corner to a quarter of the way in. Use a sponge-tipped brush to smudge the color two-thirds of the way towards the inner corner.

Tilt your head back and apply BLACK MASCARA in an upwards motion, wiggling the wand as you go. You will need several coats. Allow to dry in between each coat and keep adding until you get the ultra batty eyelashes.

Thirty minutes later you'll be ready to go out!

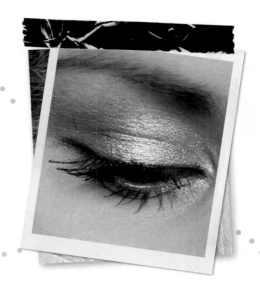

4. Apply foundation to the lips as a MATTE BASE—you will have some left over on your foundation brush.

Then apply a pale silvery-pink lipstick. Add a touch of light pink pearly lip gloss on the lower lip and the middle of the top lip.

Finish with a dab of white frosted eyeshadow in the center of the lower lip.

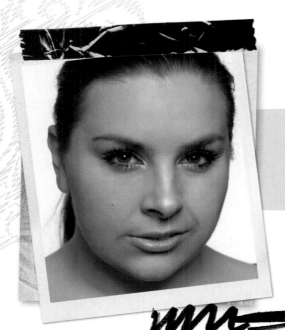

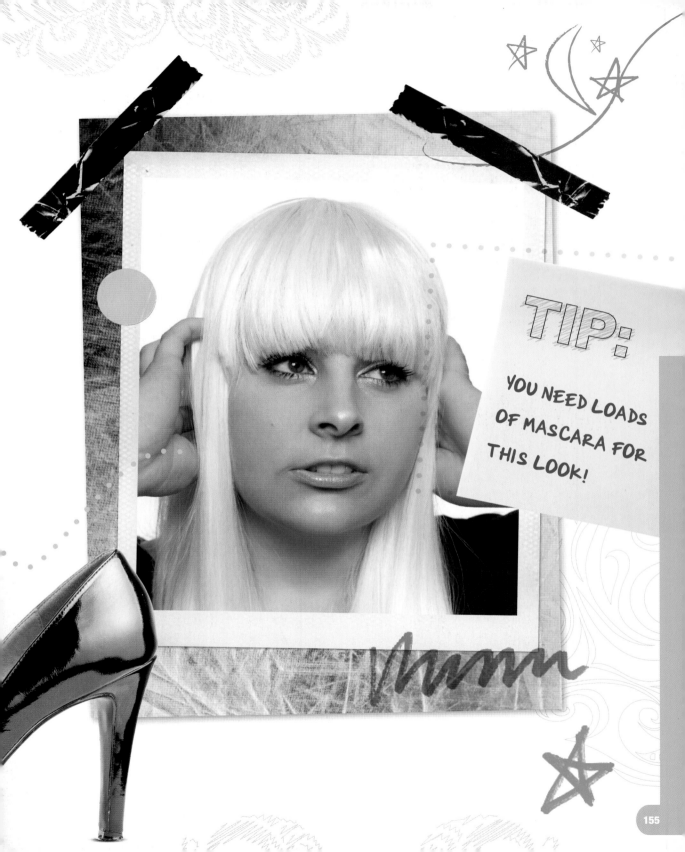

TIP:

YOU NEED LOADS OF MASCARA FOR THIS LOOK!

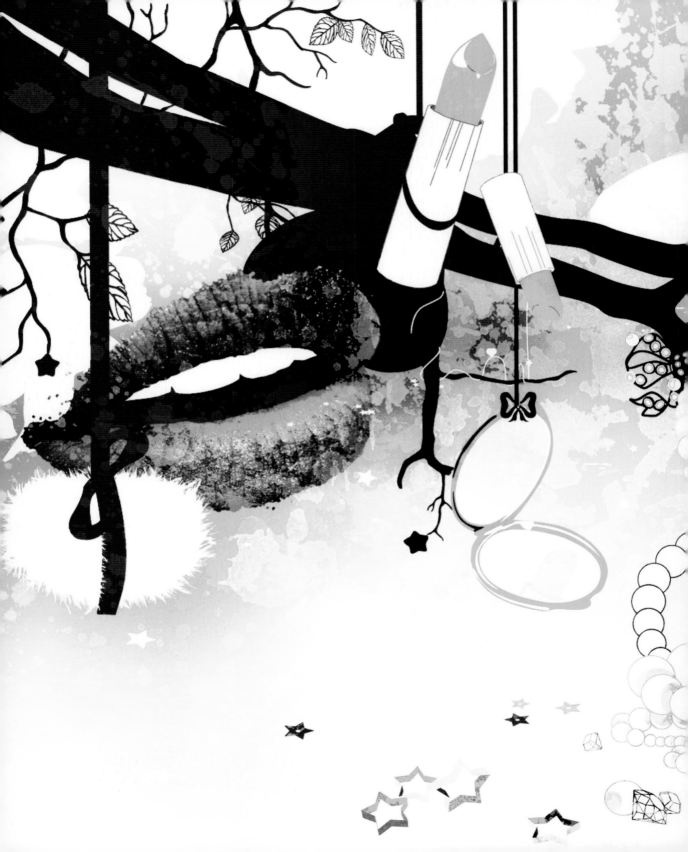

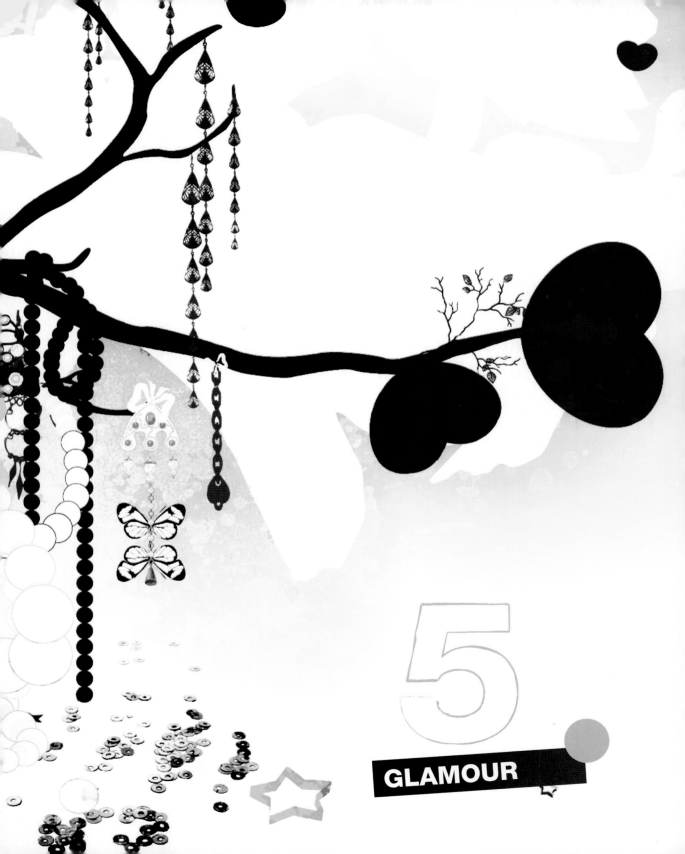

5

GLAMOUR

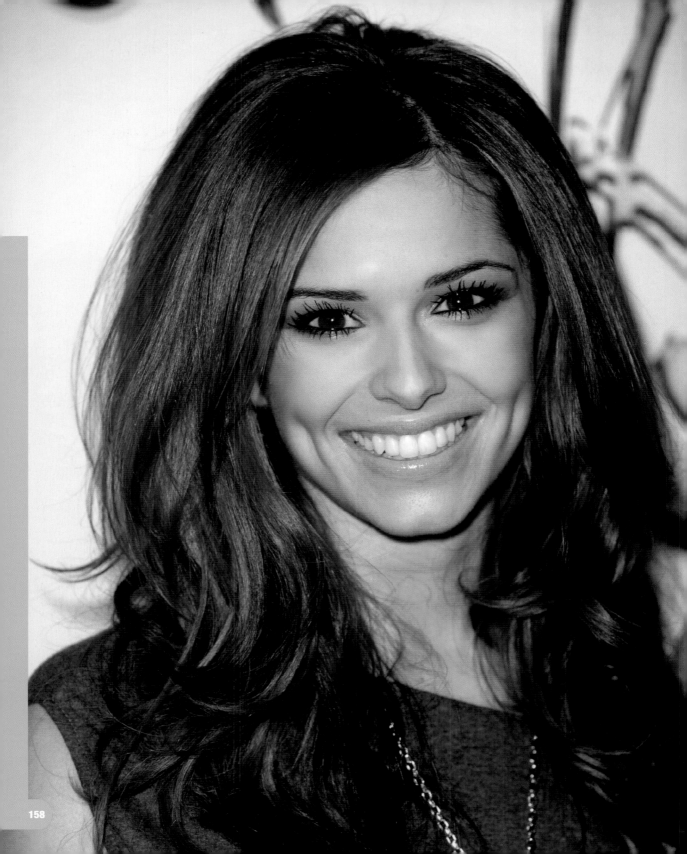

CHERYL COLE

COVER GIRL

CHERYL COLE IS EVERYONE'S FAVORITE COVER GIRL. SHE'S A FELLOW GEORDIE, AND SHE LOOKS GORGEOUS. THIS IS ANOTHER DARK, SPARKLY LOOK, BUT THIS TIME IT'S BRONZED AND SUN KISSED.

THE PALETTE

* Beige eye primer
* Light taupe frosted eye mousse
* Black frosted eyeshadow
* Pale apricot-beige frosted blush
* Deep peach frosted blush
* Black mascara
* Nude-peach lip liner pencil
* Creamy tea-colored satin lipstick
* Pearly white lip gloss

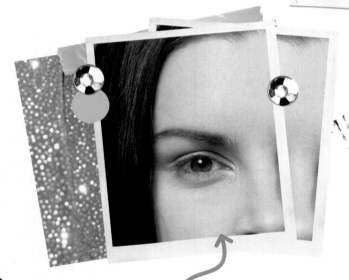

1. Use your third finger to apply a beige eye primer all over the eyelid and up to just under the eyebrow.

Apply a light taupe frosted eye mousse with your third finger, over the primer, up to the eyebrow.

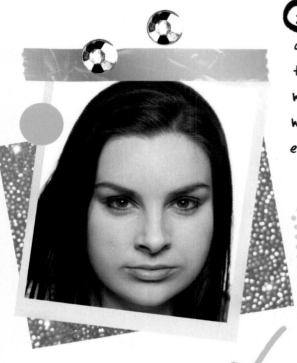

2. Use an angled eyeliner brush to apply black frosted eyeshadow along the upper lash line. Smudge the color with a blending brush so you end up with a subtle effect that covers the eyelid only, not above it.

Dampen the angled eyeliner brush and apply the black frosted eyeshadow along the lower lash line, gently dabbing the color from the outer to the inner corner. Blend well.

Then, to further darken the eye, trace a line along the outer quarter of the upper eyelid and join at the outer corner.

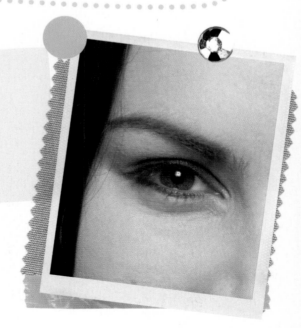

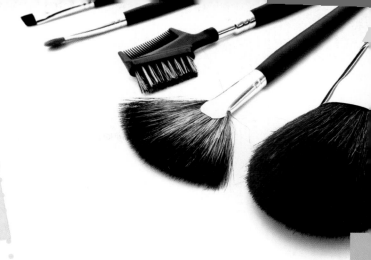

TIP:

IF THERE IS A CERTAIN EYESHADOW COLOR YOU ADORE, BUT IT DOESN'T QUITE SUIT YOUR COLORING, TRY IT WITH COLORS THAT DO. NO COLORS ARE OFF-LIMITS!

3. Using a kabuki brush, apply a pale apricot-beige frosted blush on and around the cheekbone, going right down to the jawline and just beneath.

Use the same brush to apply a deep peach blush. Smile, and follow the line from the outer lip to the ear—a straight line that entirely covers the apple of the cheek.

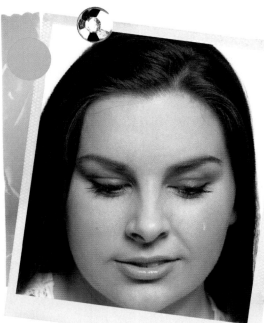

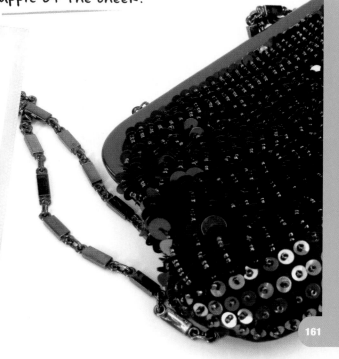

161

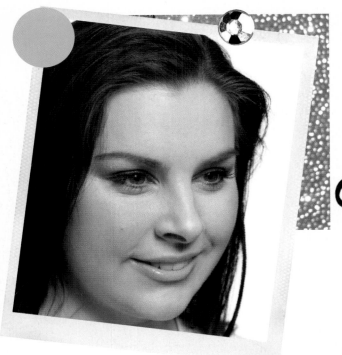

4. Tilt your head back and apply black mascara in an upward and outward motion onto the upper lashes. Allow to dry and apply a second layer.

Add a light touch of mascara to the lower lashes.

Use a creamy nude-peach lip liner pencil to trace the lip line. Fill in with a creamy tea-colored satin lipstick.

Finish with a pearly white lip gloss on the bottom lip only.

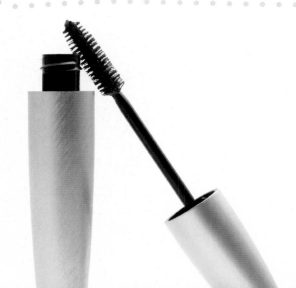

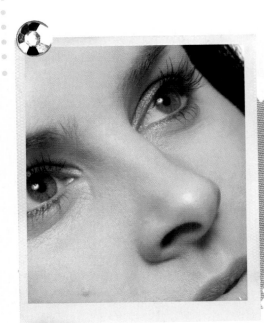

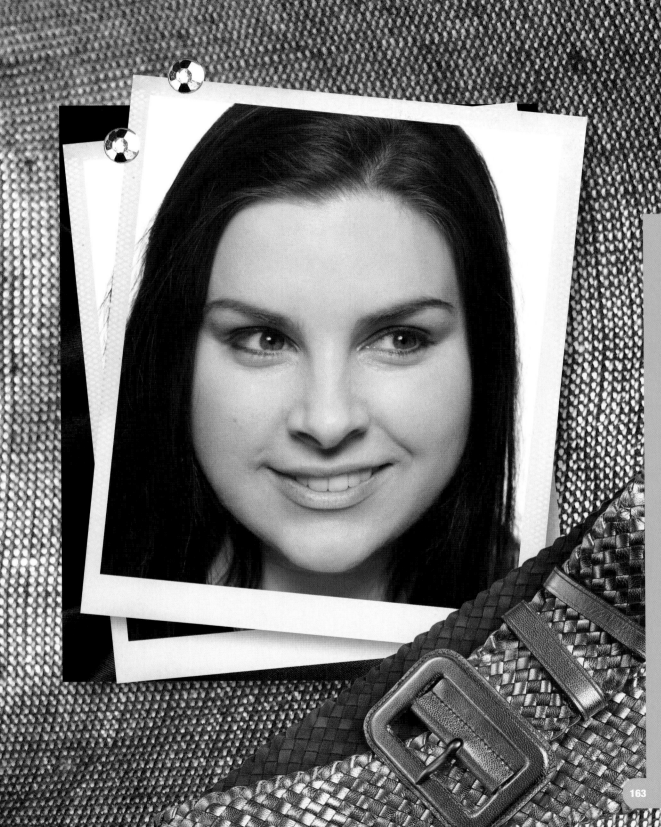

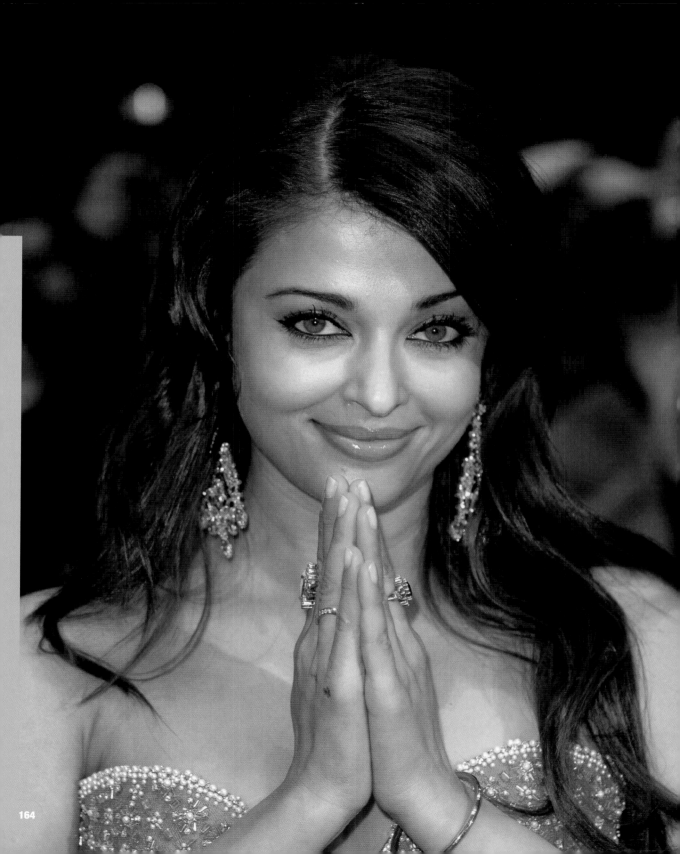

BOLLYWOOD BABY

SHE'S A STAR

BOLLYWOOD IS ALL ABOUT GLAMOUR. THINK OF THE VIBRANT, RICH, LUXURIOUS JEWEL COLORS ON AISHWARYA RAI, AND YOU WON'T FAIL WITH THIS LOOK. YOU DON'T HAVE TO FOLLOW THESE COLORS EXACTLY EITHER— EXPERIMENT.

THE PALETTE

* Beige eye primer
* Metallic gold powder eyeshadow
* Dark damson-red eyeshadow
* White pearlescent eyeshadow
* Black liquid eyeliner
* Black eyeliner pencil
* Dark plum blush
* Tea-colored matte lip pencil
* Black mascara
* Eyebrow gel
* Dark brown eyeshadow

1. Start by applying a beige eye primer with your third finger, all over the eyelid and right up to the brow bone.

THEN RUN YOUR FINGER UNDERNEATH THE EYE AS WELL.

Using an eyeshadow brush, apply a metallic gold eyeshadow powder all over the eyelid, right into the inner corner and out along the crease, extending slightly at the outer corner.

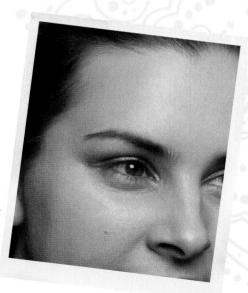

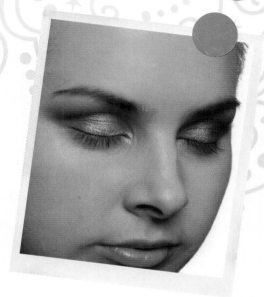

2. Tilt the head back. Using a blending brush, gently feather the damson eyeshadow just above the crease, emphasizing the outer half and fading the color towards the inner eye. BLEND WELL.

The darkness is for the outer corner, to give depth.

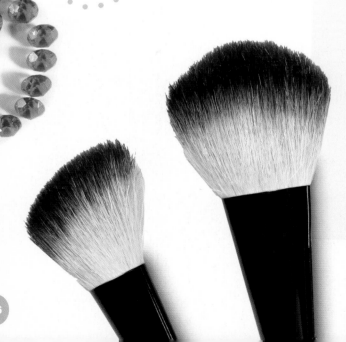

3. Dip an eyeshadow brush into white pearlescent eyeshadow and gently dab onto the brow bone, then move the brush back and forth to blend the colors.

Then, using the edge of the brush only, run the white eyeshadow along the inside of the nose, up to meet the color on the brow bone.

Blend in well, so the colors merge where they meet and soften any harsh lines.

4. With a light touch, use a black liquid eyeliner to draw a line from the center of the upper eye to the outer corner, extending a generous "wing" at the outer corner. Then work from the center to the inner corner.

Starting at the outer corner, use a black creamy eyeliner pencil along the lower lash line and into the water line (see page 29), working from the "wing" to the inner corner in a fairly thick line.

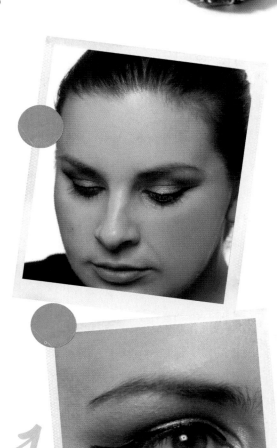

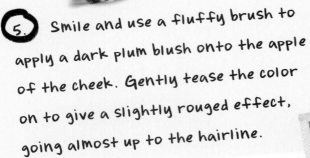

5. Smile and use a fluffy brush to apply a dark plum blush onto the apple of the cheek. Gently tease the color on to give a slightly rouged effect, going almost up to the hairline.

You want light lips for this look. Draw a line around your lips with a tea-colored matte lip pencil. Fill in the rest of your lips with the pencil

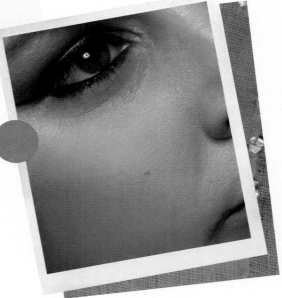

TIP:

GENTLY TEASE THE BLUSH ONTO THE CHEEK TO GIVE A SLIGHTLY ROUGED EFFECT.

6. Tilt your head back and apply black mascara, wiggling the wand as you go from the base of the lashes in and upwards and outwards motion. Leave to dry while you do the eyebrows before you apply a second coat.

Put a little eyebrow gel onto the back of your hand. Dip a squared eyeliner brush into the gel and then into a dark brown eyeshadow and apply the color to the eyebrows, flicking the brush upwards on the inner brow, squaring the arch, and tapering at the end.

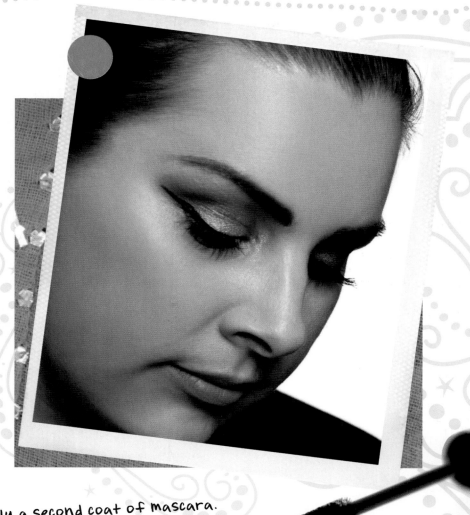

Apply a second coat of mascara.
The more dramatic the better.
Apply a little to the bottom lashes.

IF YOU HAVE FALSE EYELASHES, NOW IS THE TIME TO POP THEM ON, GIRLS.

WHEN EXPERIMENT
MAKEUP LOOKS, I
YOU MAKE MIST
AND START AG
REMEMBER, RO

NG WITH DIFFERENT
DOESN'T MATTER IF
ES. TAKE YOUR TIME
N UNTIL YOU'RE HAPPY.
E WASN'T BUILT IN A DAY.

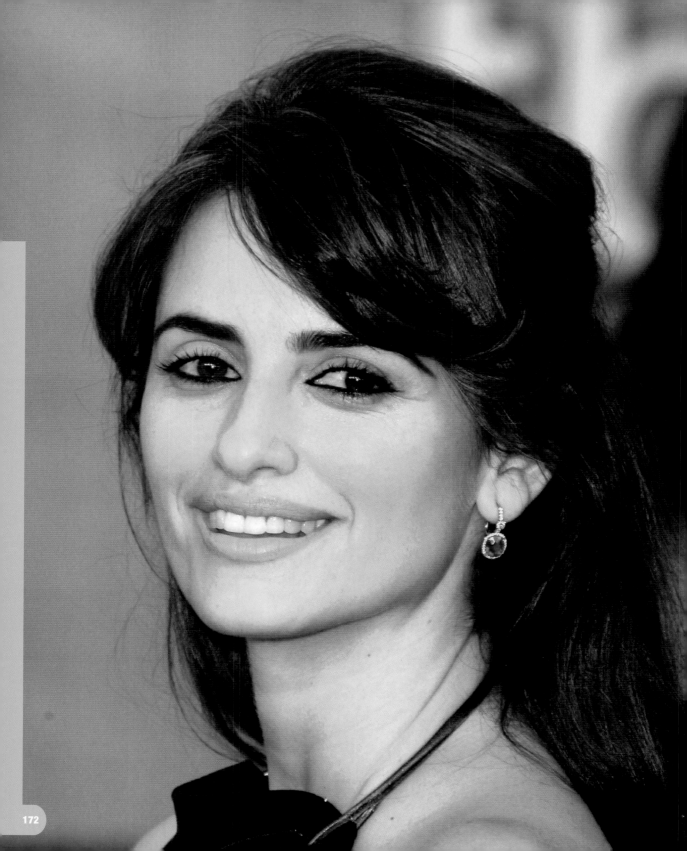

PENÉLOPE CRUZ
BELLE OF THE BALL

A NEUTRAL LOOK WITH A 1960s TWIST. THICK EYELINER ON THE UPPER LASHES, VERY STRONG EYEBROWS, AND FABULOUS, GLOSSY HAIR.

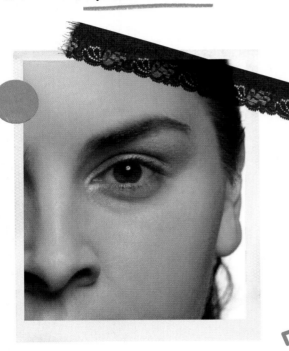

1. Start with an ivory frosted eyeshadow and apply with an eyeshadow brush all over the eyelid, patting it on right up to the brow.

Use a fluffy brush to apply a light golden matte bronzer, sweeping up and down from just under the cheekbone to the jawline. Follow this line to the hairline. Then gently feather what is left on the brush on the temples.

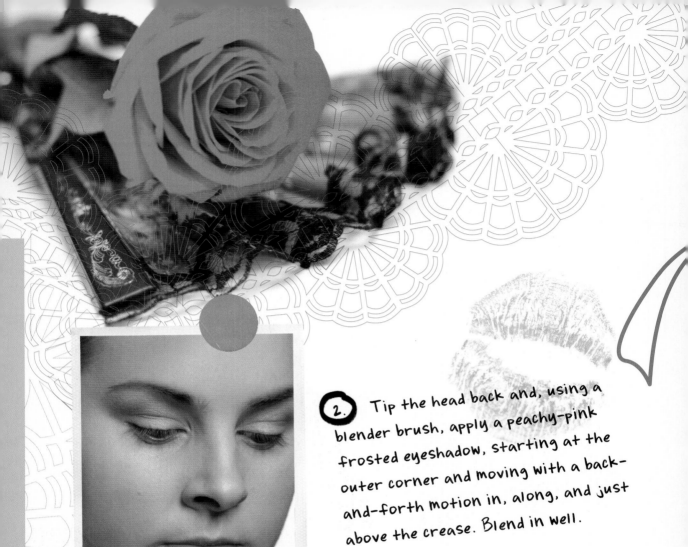

2. Tip the head back and, using a blender brush, apply a peachy-pink frosted eyeshadow, starting at the outer corner and moving with a back-and-forth motion in, along, and just above the crease. Blend in well.

Use a fluffy brush to apply a pink pearlescent highlighter. Start in the middle of the forehead and bring it down between the eyebrows onto the nose, and gently feather it from the top of the cheekbone to the hairline just above the ear. You are following and going above the bronzer line. Blend a little way down towards the edge of the nose and take it onto the chin and underneath.

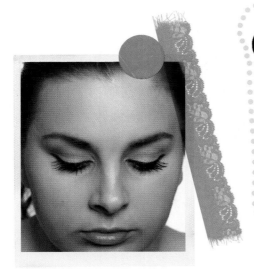

3. Gently draw a line with a black creamy eyeliner pencil from halfway across the upper eyelid to the outer corner and slightly beyond. You will be going straight out, not up in a tick. Then take the line from the inner corner to meet in the middle.

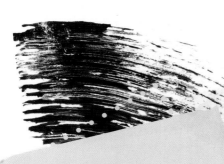

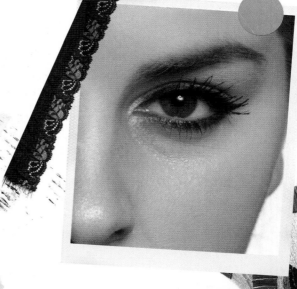

TIP: THIS WAY OF HIGHLIGHTING CREATES A 3-D EFFECT AND GIVES THE IMPRESSION OF HAVING CHEEKBONES—EVEN IF YOU DON'T.

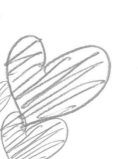

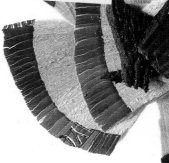

Next draw a line from the outer corner, halfway in along the lower lash line. Use a foam-tipped brush to smudge the color and blend it into the inner corner.

Use the same brush to run a little dirty gold eyeshadow over the black, on the bottom lash line only—to soften the black.

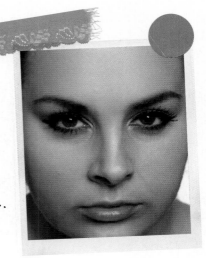

4. The eyebrows are very prominent for this look. Dip an eyebrow brush into eyebrow wax and run it up and then across the eyebrows to set them in position. Then, using the same brush and a dark brown eyebrow powder, apply the color first up and then across the brow, feathering it to the arch and then beyond. You should end up with a beautifully curved eyebrow.

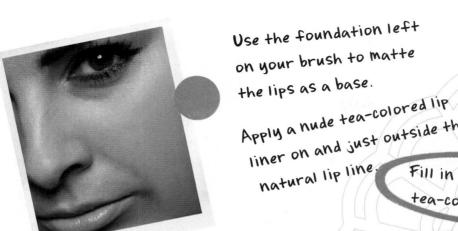

Use the foundation left on your brush to matte the lips as a base.

Apply a nude tea-colored lip liner on and just outside the natural lip line.

Fill in with a pale tea-colored lipstick.

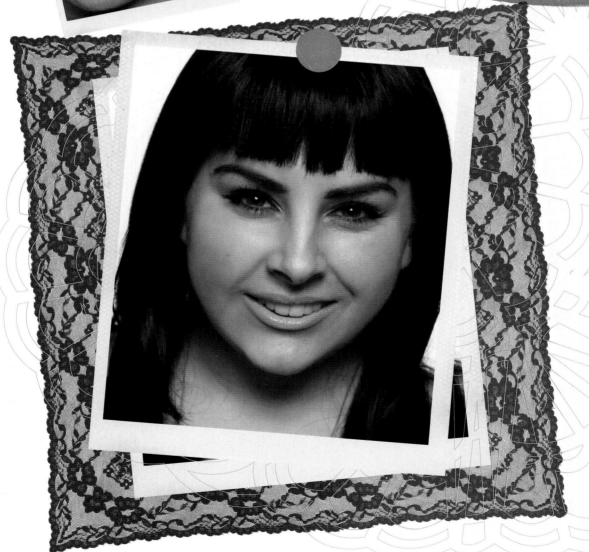

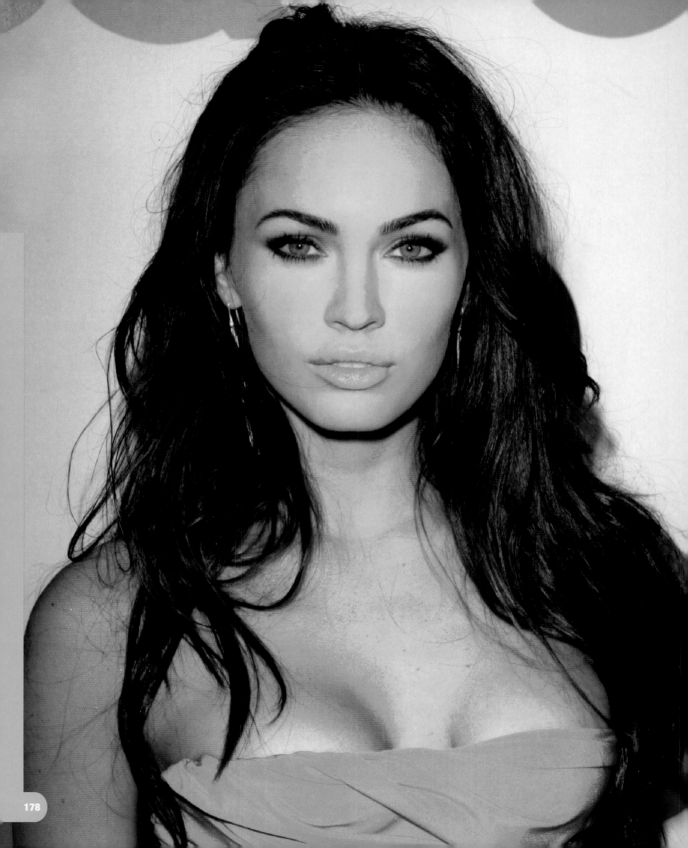

MEGAN FOX
HOT PINK

THIS IS A MOSTLY BRONZER, LIPS, AND THICK LASHES. IT'S FRESH AND PRETTY WITH A GOLDEN GLOW.

THE PALETTE

* Peachy-pink bronzer
* Beige eye primer
* Black eyeliner pencil
* Black mascara
* Eyebrow wax
* Dark brown eyebrow powder
* Nude-peach lip liner
* Light peach shimmery lip gloss

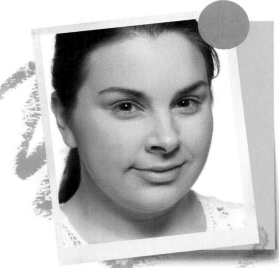

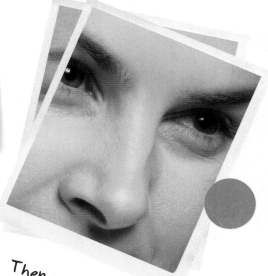

1. Start with a peachy-pink bronzer, and dab it on with a fluffy brush in a 3 motion, from the temple, round to the cheekbone, and down under the jawline.

Then run the brush down the nose with a touch on the chin.

179

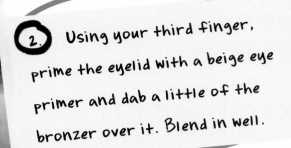

2. Using your third finger, prime the eyelid with a beige eye primer and dab a little of the bronzer over it. Blend in well.

Using a black creamy eyeliner pencil, tight line (see page 30) the outer half of the upper eyelid, and do the same on the water line (see page 29) of the lower eyelid.

Using the same pencil, draw a line from the middle of the upper eyelid to just beyond the outer corner. Use a sponge-tipped eyeliner brush to smudge the color and smooth it towards the inner corner, staying very close to the lashes.

3. Tilt your head back and apply thick, thick black mascara. Keep putting on extra coats until you are happy—I've done three layers, building up the thickness each time. Apply on bottom lashes as well.

Use a squared eyeliner brush to apply eyebrow wax in a stroking motion along the eyebrows.

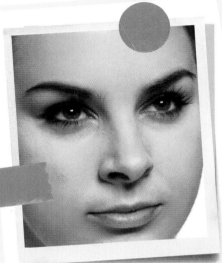

TIP:

YOU WANT THE EYELASHES TO BE SHORT AND CHUNKY RATHER THAN LONG AND THIN FOR THIS LOOK.

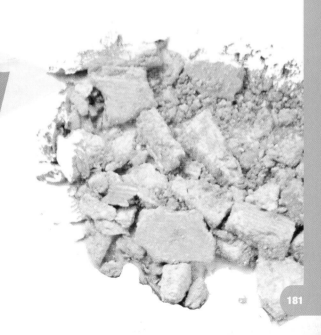

Dab the brush in dark brown eyebrow powder and apply to the brows to give a really dark, shiny look.

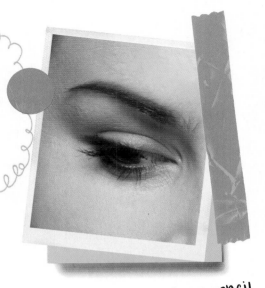

4. Take a nude-peach matte lip liner pencil to trace the lips. The color shouldn't be too strong because you will not be using lipstick, only lip gloss, over the lip liner.

Use a light peach shimmery lip gloss to blend with the lip liner and fill in the lips.

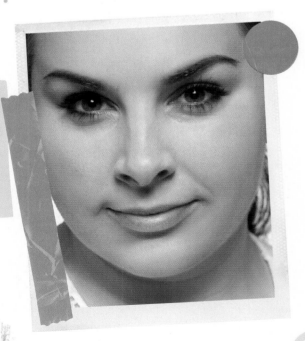

TIP:

SMILING IS VERY INFECTIOUS, GIVE IT A GO AND SMILE AT PEOPLE AS YOU WALK BY. YOU'LL BE SURPRISED BY HOW MANY PEOPLE SMILE BACK AND THE UPLIFTING FEELING YOU GET IN RETURN.

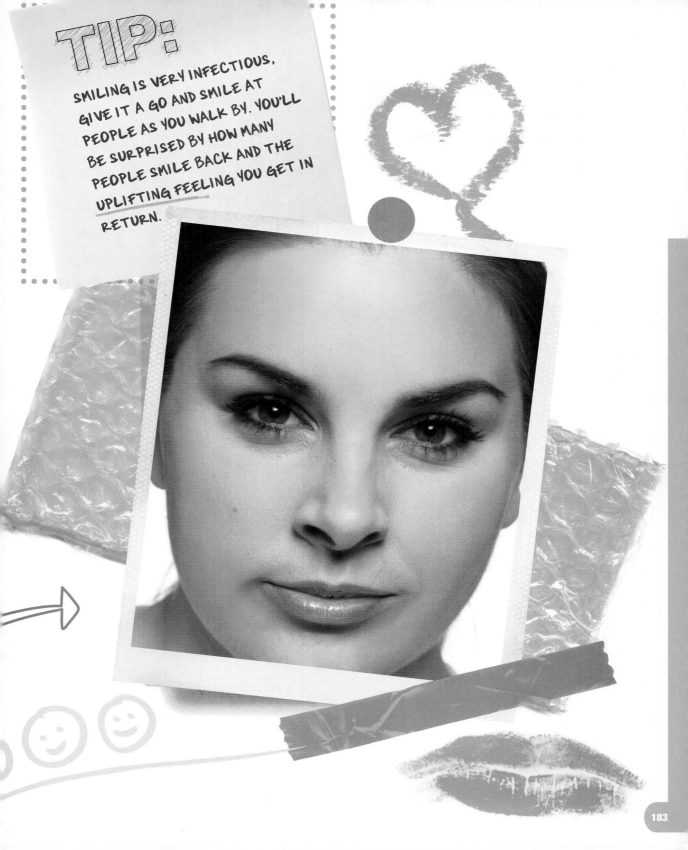

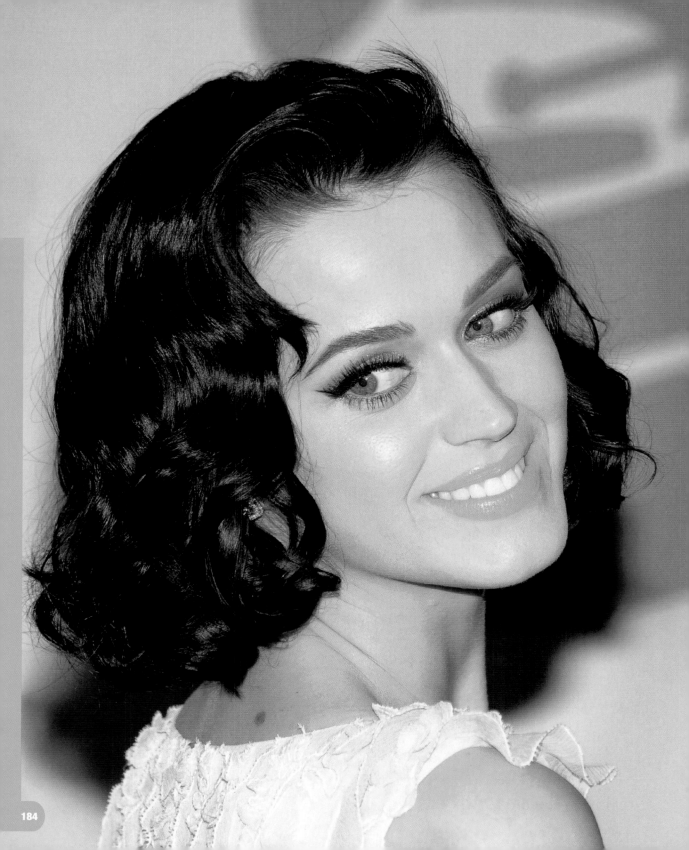

KATY PERRY

CASINO GLAMOUR

I LOVE KATY'S KITSCH GLAMOUR LOOK—IT'S VERY GLAM. HERE IS HER "WAKING UP IN VEGAS" LOOK— SILVER WITH SMOKY BLACK EYES AND NUDE-PEACH LIPS.

THE PALETTE

* White frosted eyeshadow
* Silver eyeshadow powder
* Eyebrow gel
* Black frosted eyeshadow
* Black liquid eyeliner
* Black mascara
* Golden apricot bronzer
* Golden terra-cotta frosted lipstick
* Nude shimmery lip gloss

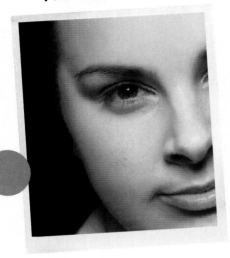

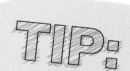

TIP:

THE WHITE FROSTED EYESHADOW HIGHLIGHTS THE SILVER AND GIVES IT THAT EXTRA ZING.

1. Prime the eyes with white frosted eyeshadow, using your third finger to go over the eyelid and up to the eyebrow.

   Using an eyeshadow brush, apply silver eyeshadow powder all over the eyelid to just above the crease.

   Gently dab a little more in the center of the eyelid. Then add a little white frosted eyeshadow on top as a highlight.

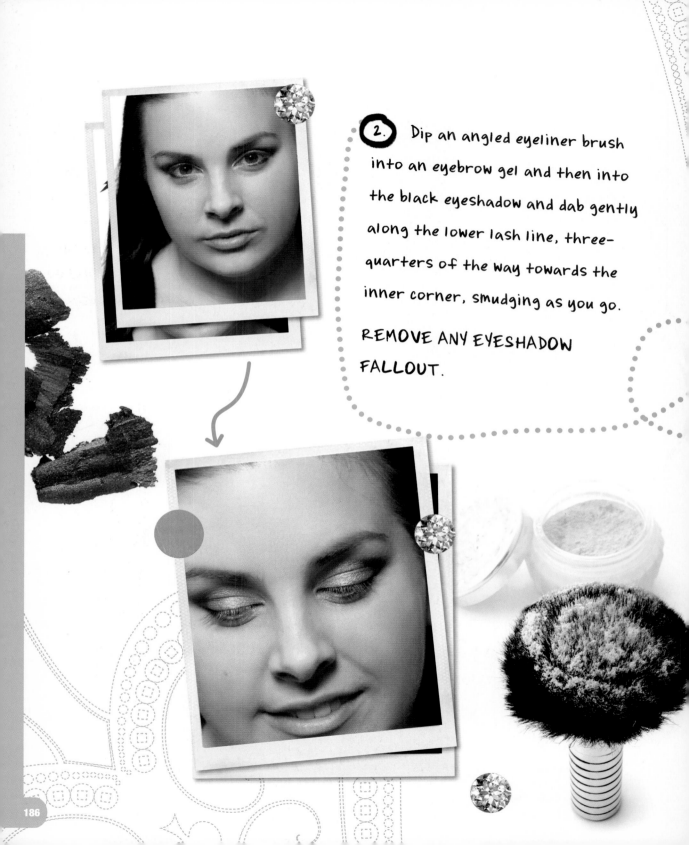

2. Dip an angled eyeliner brush into an eyebrow gel and then into the black eyeshadow and dab gently along the lower lash line, three-quarters of the way towards the inner corner, smudging as you go.

REMOVE ANY EYESHADOW FALLOUT.

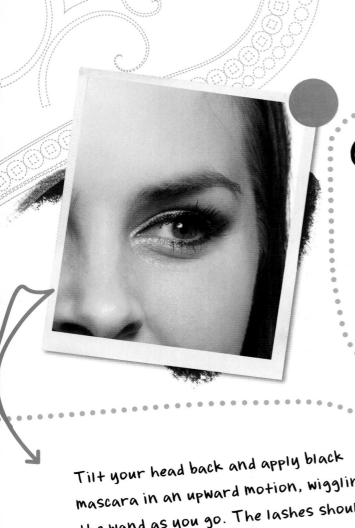

3. Using the same brush, apply black liquid eyeliner from the middle of the upper eyelid to the outer corner. Then apply from the inner corner to join the line in the middle. It should be a very fine line, as close to the lashes as possible.

Tilt your head back and apply black mascara in an upward motion, wiggling the wand as you go. The lashes should be thick and full.

Add a touch of mascara to the lower lashes.

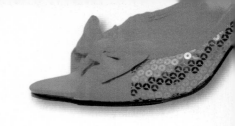

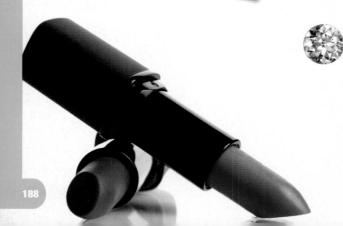

4. Using a fluffy brush and starting one brush width out from the lower lip, gently waft a golden apricot bronzer on and below the cheekbone going up to meet the hairline at the top of the ear. Work the color in well.

Apply a golden terra-cotta frosted lipstick to the top and bottom lips.

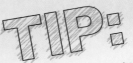

TAME THE COLOR WITH A LITTLE NUDE SHIMMERY LIP GLOSS.

TIP:

GET AS MUCH HANDS-ON EXPERIENCES AS YOU CAN— PRACTICE ON YOUR OWN FACE OR ANYONE ELSE'S FACE YOU CAN GRAB FOR A MAKEOVER—YOU'LL FEEL MUCH MORE CONFIDENT AND LEARN NEW TECHNIQUES.

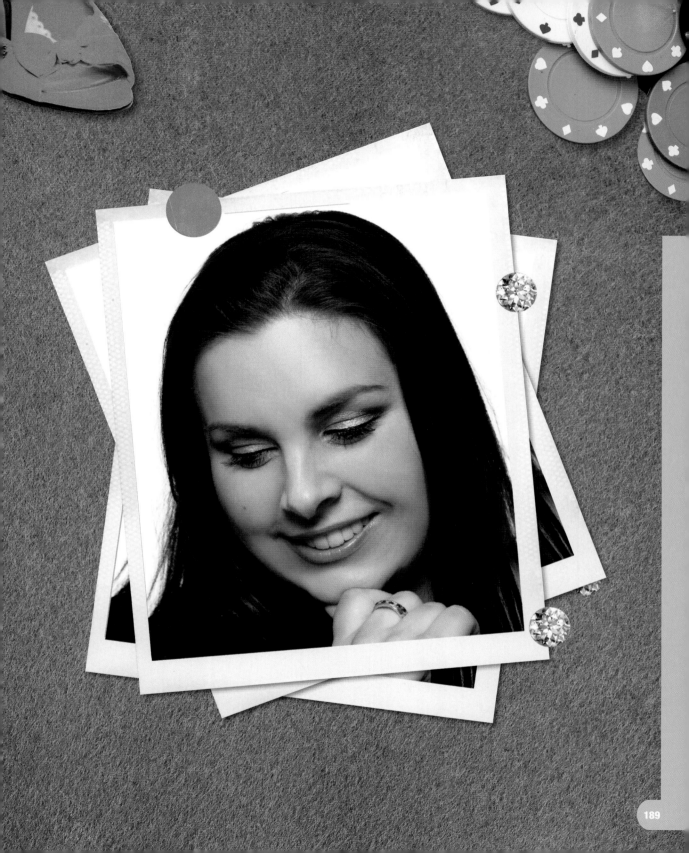

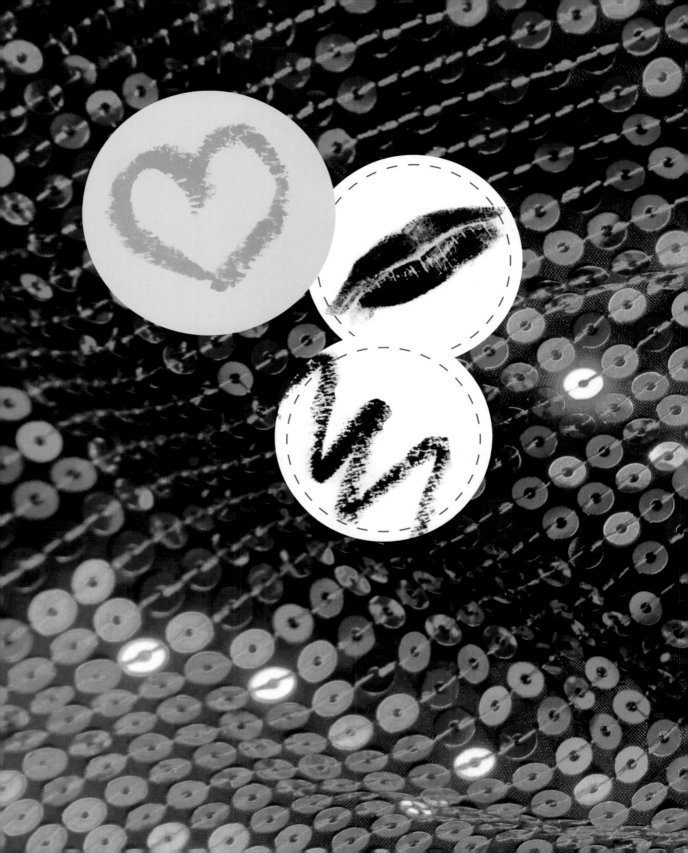

A NIGHT OUT IS A REAL OPPORTUNITY TO BE MORE IMAGINATIVE AND CREATIVE WITH YOUR MAKEUP. DON'T BE SCARED—WEAR WHATEVER YOU LIKE AND BE MORE FREE WITH YOUR LOOK— IT'S A TIME TO LET YOUR PERSONALITY SHOW.

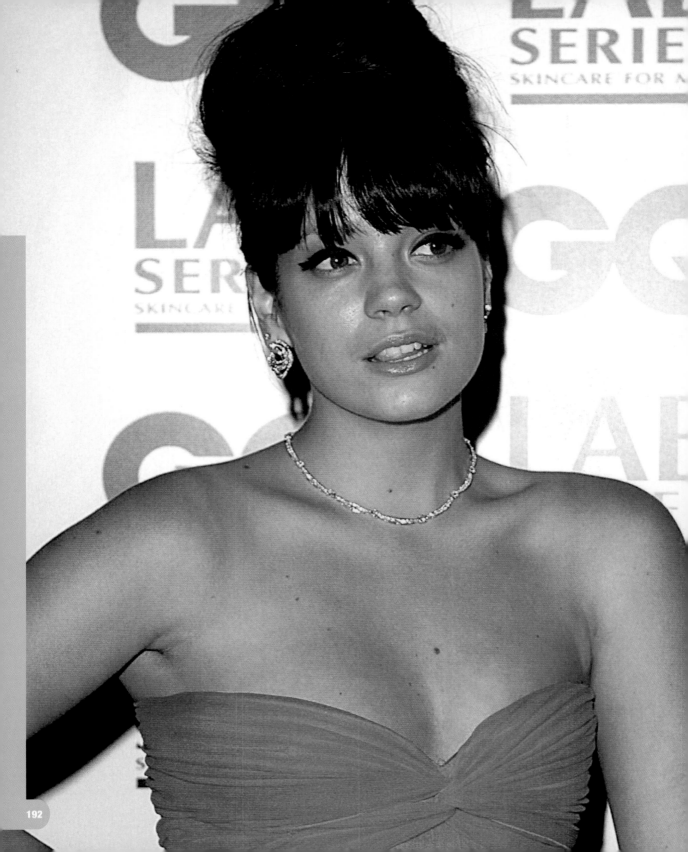

LILY ALLEN

ROCK GODDESS

A DEEP, DARK, SMOKY GREEN
LOOK ADDS MYSTERY TO THE EYES.
IF THEY ARE THE WINDOWS
TO SOUL, HE'S NOT GOING TO
BE ABLE TO STOP LOOKING
DEEP INTO YOURS.

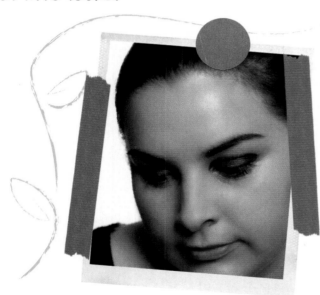

THE PALETTE

* Beige frosted eye primer
* Dark green frosted eyeshadow
* Black liquid eyeliner
* Black creamy eyeliner pencil
* Peach frosted eyeshadow
* Black mascara
* Peachy-pink matte blush
* Tea-colored lip liner
* Tea-colored satin lipstick
* Ivory-pink lip gloss

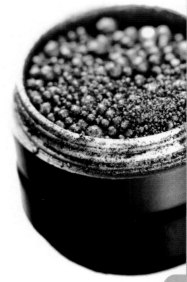

1. Use your third finger to apply a beige frosted eye primer all over the eyelid and up to the eyebrow. Give it a good coating.

   Using an eyeshadow brush, apply dark green frosted eyeshadow all over the eyelid, up to the crease and a little way past it. Do not extend the color at the outer edge.

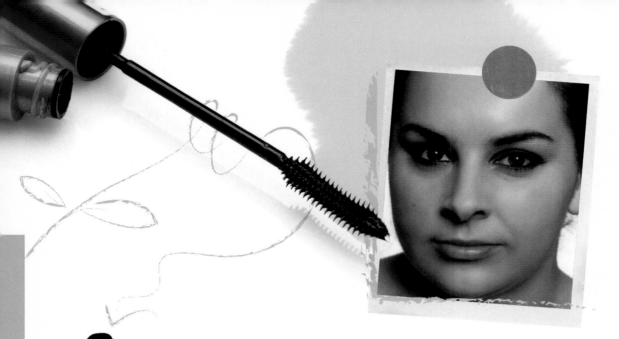

2. Starting halfway across the upper eyelid, use a black liquid eyeliner to draw a fine line to the outer edge, finishing with a tiny tick (use an angled eyeliner brush instead of the applicator—it can be tricky). Then draw a line from the inner corner to meet in the middle.

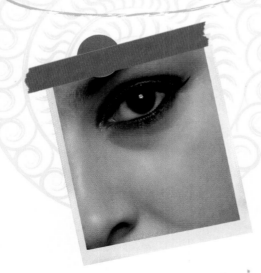

Use a black creamy eyeliner pencil to gently draw a line along the lower lash line from the outer corner halfway in. Use a sponge-tipped brush to smudge the color into the inner corner. Then apply to the water line (see page 29) as well.

3. With a blender brush run a peach frosted eyeshadow lightly over the crease, back and forth, on top of the green. The color should be barely visible.

TIP:
EXPERIMENT WITH MAKEUP WHEN YOU HAVE A CLEAR TIME SLOT. SET SOME TIME ASIDE AND DON'T RUSH IT—YOU'LL LEARN AND PROGRESS MORE. AND MOST IMPORTANTLY, YOU'LL ENJOY IT!

Apply black mascara in an upwards motion, wiggling the wand as you go. Allow to dry and apply a second coat.

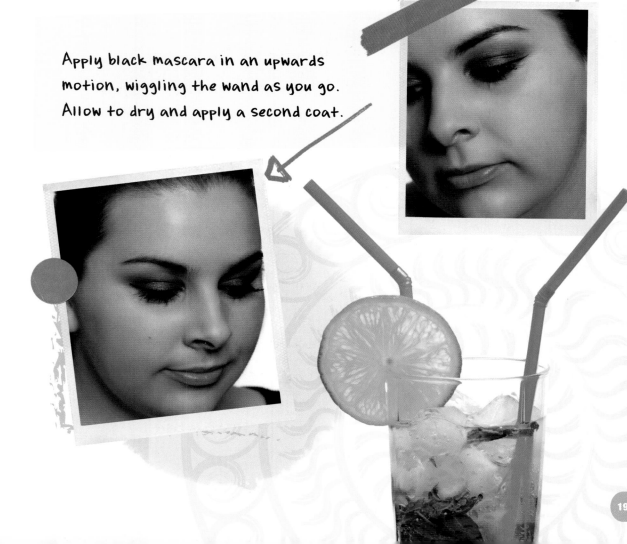

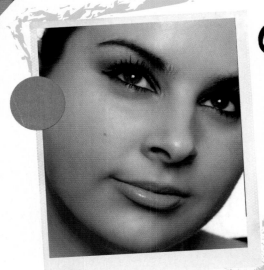

4. Make a fish face. **Using a** kabuki brush, apply a peachy-pink matte blush from under the apple of the cheek in a straight line up to the hairline. Blend in with a back-and-forth motion.

Run a nude, tea-colored lip liner around the natural lip line and slightly beyond the edges.

Fill in with a tea-colored satin lipstick.

Finish with an ivory-pink lip gloss.

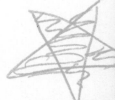

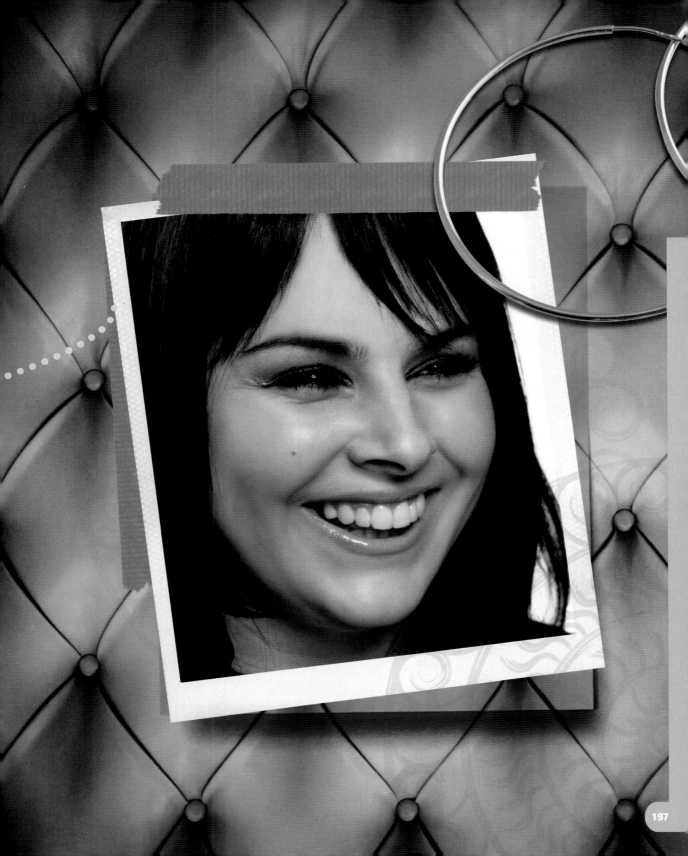

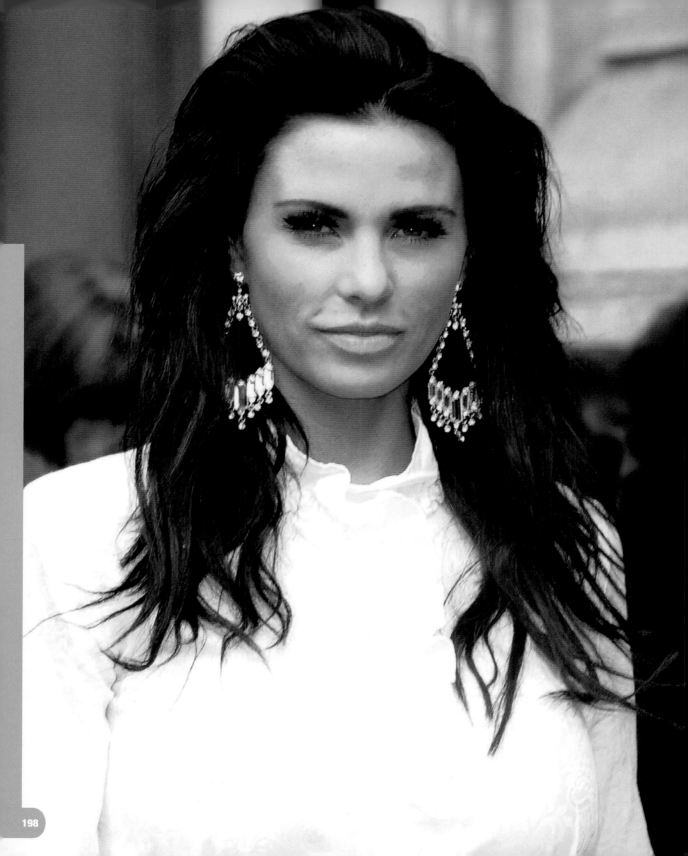

KATIE PRICE

PINUP GIRL

THIS LOOK IS PINK ON PINK WITH LAVISH LASHES. IT'S AN INCREDIBLY PRETTY LOOK AND SUITS EVERYONE.

THE PALETTE

* Beige eye primer
* Pale pink frosted eyeshadow
* White frosted eye powder
* Dark purple frosted eyeshadow
* Black liquid eyeliner
* Black creamy eyeliner pencil
* Ivory pearlescent highlighter
* Pale pink blush
* Black mascara
* Eyebrow wax
* Dark brown eyebrow powder
* Plum-pink creamy lip pencil
* Light pearly pink lipstick

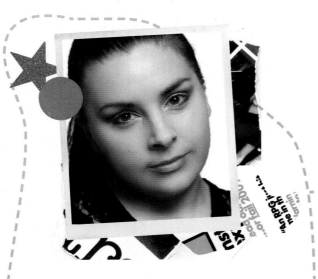

1. With your third finger, apply a beige primer all over the eyelid and up to the eyebrow, adding a little underneath the eye.

Use an eyeshadow brush to apply pale pink frosted eyeshadow all over the eyelid and just above the crease, extending slightly at the outer edge.

With the same brush, apply a tiny bit of white frosted eye powder by the inner eye, along the side of the nose, and up to the eyebrow. Blend back and forth into the pink.

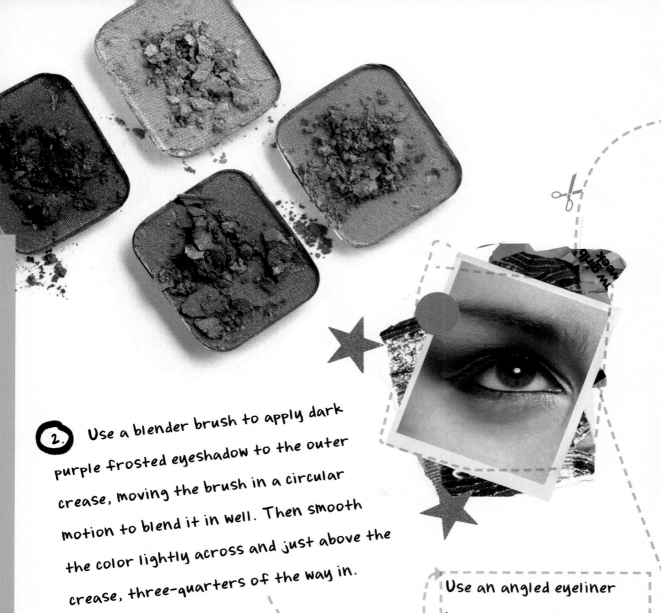

2. Use a blender brush to apply dark purple frosted eyeshadow to the outer crease, moving the brush in a circular motion to blend it in well. Then smooth the color lightly across and just above the crease, three-quarters of the way in.

Add a little more white frosted eye powder over the purple and up under the eyebrow to soften the color and give the effect of a deeper pink color rather than purple.

Use an angled eyeliner brush to feather the purple eye powder along the lower lash line from the outer corner to three-quarters of the way in.

3. Use the same brush to apply black liquid eyeliner from the middle of the upper eyelid to the outer corner. Then draw a line from the inner corner to meet in the middle.

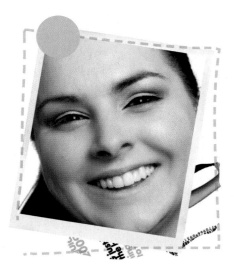

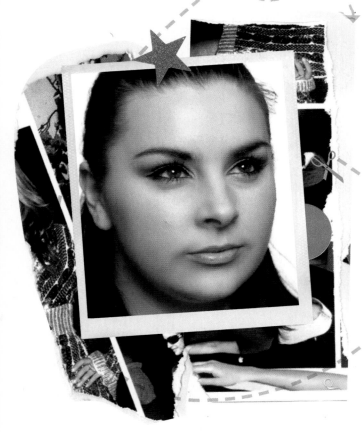

Take a black creamy eyeliner pencil and run it along the water line (see page 29) above the lower lashes.

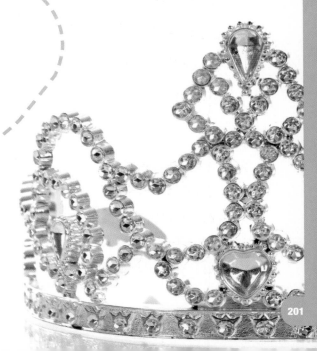

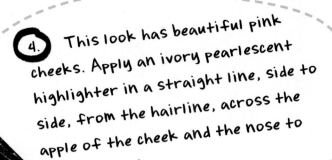

4. This look has beautiful pink cheeks. Apply an ivory pearlescent highlighter in a straight line, side to side, from the hairline, across the apple of the cheek and the nose to the other side.

Use a fluffy brush to apply a very light pale pink blusher. Gently swirl it just under the highlighter, going up to the hairline again.

5. Apply black mascara, upwards and outwards. You will need two or three layers to get the effect.

Apply mascara to the lower lashes.

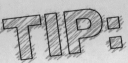

TIP:

DON'T WEAR CLOTHES OR MAKEUP YOU DON'T FEEL COMFORTABLE IN JUST BECAUSE A MAGAZINE TELLS YOU TO. JUST CHOOSE THE THINGS THAT MAKE YOU FEEL GOOD.

Use a squared eyeliner brush to apply eyebrow wax and to make a rounded shape. Use the same brush to tease dark brown eyebrow powder through the eyebrow to enhance the shape.

Now add another coat of mascara to thicken the lashes.

6. The lips should be really pouty. Use a plum-pink creamy lip pencil to draw a line around and just outside the natural lip line, crossing over the Cupid's bow and tapering in at

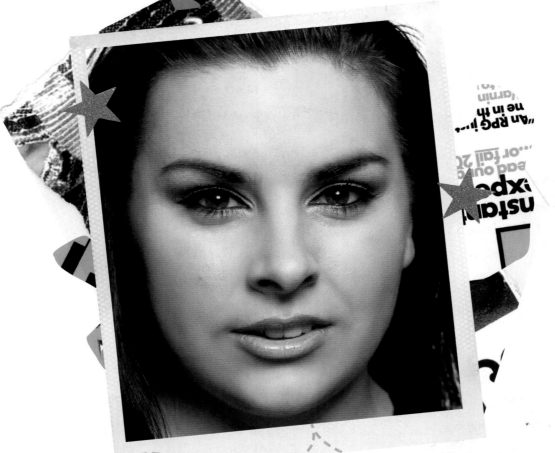

Then fill the lips in with a light, pearly-pink lipstick.

How do I get rid of spots?

I've been told of two ways to deal with spots. As soon as you wake up—before you've had a drink or anything to eat—lick a finger and dab it around the spot that you can feel coming on. The bacteria that accumulates in your mouth overnight will do wonders for zapping the spot!

Or, if you're not too keen on the dragon's breath method, try tea tree oil. Lick a finger first, add a drop of oil, and apply to the spot—you'll see rapid results.

My eyes are hidden behind my glasses. Can you make my eyes pop with a neutral look?

Start with a matte finish eyeshadow in ivory or cream. Apply all over the eyelid to just past the crease.

Take a frosted chocolate-brown eyeshadow and apply to the outer crease and just above to give the eyes a little depth. Then take an eyeshadow that is a similar color to your eyebrows and gently tease the color onto the eyebrow to give a stronger shape.

Use a black liquid eyeliner to make a very thin line all the way across the upper lashes. Gently smudge the chocolate-brown eyeshadow along the outer quarter of the lower lash line.

Apply only a little mascara—so the lashes don't look spidery. And voilà, people will see your eyes instead of the glasses.

Is it safe to use mascaras that are several months old? They have hardly been used.

Because eyes are such a sensitive area, it's best not to take the chance. Regardless of how many times it has been used, if it's past five months old, you definitely need to put it in the bin. Try and refresh your mascara every four or five months, max, to keep your eyelashes in good shape.

What is the quickest way to remove a mascara smudge?

Wait until the mascara has dried and wipe it off with a Q-tip. It should come off easily. You will be less likely to catch your skin in the first place if you tilt your head back to apply the mascara.

One of my eyes is larger than the other. How can I make them look equal?

Apply a light-colored eyeshadow equally on each side, taking it up to the eyebrow. Take a darker-colored eyeshadow and apply to both creases, applying a little more to the side that's bigger. Blend well. If you are using liquid eyeliner on the upper lash line, make it slightly thicker on the bigger eye. ☺

Can you please give me tips on how to apply eyeliner? I always blink and my hands shake a lot.

It's a natural reflex to blink when you have something pointed at your eyeball. This happened to me when I started—and I would panic about blinking to the point it would make me blink and I wouldn't want to try again. But be patient—you'll get the hang of it in no time.

Steady your hand by resting your little finger on the cheekbone. Start with a gel liner that you apply with a long, angled eyeliner brush. Gently pull the skin taut to keep it nice and smooth and stop the eye from moving. Stop, blink, and go back to it.

You can take as long as you need on this—it's not something to be done in a flash.

You are really talented— YOU'RE AN ARTIST!

I have small eyes. How do I wear liquid eyeliner?

Make a line along your upper lashes as usual, and as you get to the outer corner thicken the line a little and lift it with a slight flick.

Use a creamy black eyeliner pencil along the lower lash line. Start from the outer corner and gently smudge it inwards, making sure the line is thicker at the outer corner and thinner as you move towards the inner eye.

Take a creamy white eyeliner pencil and apply all over the water line, starting from the outer corner and working in. Take it right to the inner corner, and then onto the upper water line. This will really open up your eyes.

What makeup should I wear with a red dress that has silver trim on the neckline?

Use a sparkly silver eyeshadow, a tiny line of black eyeliner along the upper lashes, and a red stained effect on the lips (apply the lipstick with a finger). These colors also look good if you are wearing black or white.